Critical Thinking Skills for Healthcare

Thinking critically is an essential skill, both for students and for the modern, evidence-based, healthcare practitioner. You need to be able to find, understand and evaluate the evidence that underpins your assignments, clinical decision making and practice. The good news is that you use all of these skills in everyday life. You don't believe every advert you see or respond to every spam email. It's just a question of taking these critical skills and having the confidence to apply them to your academic work. This book will help you do just that. It will enable you to:

- recognise your existing ability to be a critical thinker
- spot logical flaws and inconsistencies in arguments
- consider health issues from multiple perspectives, weighing up the strengths and weaknesses of a case
- build a convincing argument in assessments
- develop a range of critical skills for successful study and healthcare practice.

Critical Thinking Skills for Healthcare is an essential resource for all health professionals in training.

Stephanie McKendry is the Widening Access Manager of the University of Strathclyde, Glasgow, UK. Previous to that she spent over twelve years in various teaching roles in higher education institutions including six years working with healthcare students.

Critical Thinking Skills for Healthcare

Stephanie McKendry

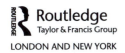
Routledge
Taylor & Francis Group

LONDON AND NEW YORK

First published 2016
by Routledge
2 Park Square, Milton Park, Abingdon, Oxon OX14 4RN

and by Routledge
711 Third Avenue, New York, NY 10017

Routledge is an imprint of the Taylor & Francis Group, an informa business

British Library Cataloguing-in-Publication Data
A catalogue record for this book is available from the British Library

Library of Congress Cataloging in Publication Data
McKendry, Stephanie, author.
Critical thinking skills for healthcare / written by Stephanie McKendry.
    p. ; cm.
  Includes bibliographical references and index.
  I. Title.
  [DNLM: 1. Clinical Competence. 2. Evidence-Based Medicine.
  3. Decision Making. 4. Health Knowledge, Attitudes, Practice.
  5. Problem-Based Learning. 6. Thinking. WB 102.5]
  RC55
  616–dc23   2015004044

ISBN: 978-1-138-78751-3 (hbk)
ISBN: 978-1-138-78752-0 (pbk)
ISBN: 978-1-315-76640-9 (ebk)

Typeset in Times
by HWA Text and Data Management, London

Printed and bound in the United States of America by Publishers Graphics,
LLC on sustainably sourced paper.

For Ross, Deb and Mam (today's critical thinkers) and
Alesia, Josie and Sadie (the next generation of critical thinkers)

Contents

Figures

Tables

Introduction

Critical thinking at university

Whatever the degree subject, upon graduating, a successful student should have developed critical thinking skills. These are the general thinking abilities that distinguish someone that has been to university. The capacity to:

- ask awkward or uncomfortable questions and not be dismissed with easy answers;
- consider issues from an objective viewpoint;
- evaluate varying perspectives before coming to a balanced judgement that can be substantiated with credible evidence.

In the early years of a degree programme, those students that can demonstrate critical thinking tend to be rewarded with the highest marks. In later years, however, it is something expected of every student as a minimum standard of ability. In dissertations, reports and essays, in fact in any assessment in the latter part of your programme, markers are looking for evidence of a critical approach. So if your essay topic is 'the inter-professional team', it isn't enough to simply describe what that is. Instead, you are expected to consider what it means for the different professions. Does it lead to effective care for patients/clients? What evidence is there for this, for example? You need to consider, argue and evaluate all aspects of the issue.

I've been working with healthcare students for over five years and I find the most common reason students don't do as well as they had hoped in assessments is because they have failed to be critical. Either they haven't understood the level of analysis and discussion expected of them, they haven't explicitly demonstrated this level within their assessment or they aren't sure how to critically examine a subject. This can be extremely frustrating for students. Often, they have spent a lot of time on the coursework and have a real knowledge of the topic so they don't understand why they have received a low mark. The problem, as I say, is a lack of criticality. The good news is that this can be remedied. It is possible to develop your critical skills and apply them to university work and professional practice.

Does any of the feedback in Box 0.1 sound familiar? Look back over past feedback and see what kind of comments your tutors have made about your work? Is there a pattern? Do you tend to always do well at the same things and regularly receive poor marks for others? Why might this be? Is there any mention of being critical?

Box 0.1 Examples of feedback

- You have been too descriptive.
- This is limited to superficial and narrow description.
- You need to be more critical.
- This is lacking in analysis.
- Why is this the case? More discussion needed here.
- Can you give an example of how this might have an impact in practice?
- More depth required.
- Why does this matter?
- What are the implications of this debate?
- You have not reached any conclusions, just presented different sides of the argument.

Critical thinking in healthcare

Healthcare degrees are particularly challenging. As well as all of the usual university learning, you are expected to uphold professional standards, undertake clinical and placement learning and acquire clinical skills. Quite understandably, the majority of students prioritise their clinical and theoretical learning (the actual content of their course and the skills they need for professional practice), but it is just as important to develop academic skills at the same time. In particular, it is essential that healthcare students acquire critical thinking skills. These are necessary to successfully complete assessments, but more than that, they are a key aspect of your professional role.

Every registered healthcare practitioner requires critical skills, for lots of reasons. For example:

1. Applying guidelines

Most health professions have clear guidelines and policies that inform their roles, duties and actions. Best practice guidelines developed by NICE (National Institute for Health and Clinical Excellence) or SIGN (Scottish Intercollegiate Guidelines Network) are adhered to by nurses, for example. It is still up to you, however, to decide which guidelines are appropriate in this particular case, with this particular client, at this particular point in your dealings with them. What will you do if circumstances change? Do the guidelines cover that or do you now need to refer to other more appropriate ones? This is where critical thinking comes in. You are not simply following a set of instructions. You are selecting guidelines, understanding the reasons behind them and applying them to the specific circumstances under which you are operating.

2. Linking theory to practice

You require critical skills to link theory to practice. Putting together the theoretical knowledge you acquire at university (the content of lectures, tutorials and your own research) with your placement learning and clinical experience is difficult. How can you relate the occasionally dry books and theories to the real-life situations you find yourself in when on placement or once registered? Conversely, how can you better understand and apply knowledge, evidence and best practice to the client scenario you are dealing with?

3. Keeping up to date with research

No matter how successful your studies, you won't have all of the knowledge you require once you graduate and register. You will continue learning throughout your professional life, undertaking professional development programmes, staying up to date with techniques and perhaps even changing your particular career focus. This will all require critical thought. So it isn't something you only need for this assessment, so that you can pass the year, graduate and get on with the real job. Critical thinking is part of the real job. Furthermore, things will change – theory, society, guidelines, scientific knowledge will all move on, often advancing rapidly. Practices that were a standard part of your undergraduate education may well be obsolete or out of date in a few years. The only way to stay current is to continue learning. It is vital you stay up to date with the latest research and that you can critically evaluate and apply it.

4. Contribute to the body of knowledge

As you become more expert in your field, you may decide to actively contribute to the evidence and knowledge that underpins practice. You might participate in research projects; you might lead them. You might undertake a systematic review and disseminate your findings at conferences or in publications. This is how progress is made and practice is improved. You will require advanced critical skills to undertake any of these tasks.

The ability to question, analyse, discuss, compare and contrast are all vital in the healthcare professions

Evidence based practice

Perhaps the most compelling reason for healthcare students to develop their critical skills is because they will be joining an evidence-based profession. You have probably encountered the concept within the course of your studies, as it is a fundamental principle for most healthcare disciplines. At its simplest, evidence-based practice is a combination of experience, expertise and available research. It is making use of all sources of knowledge (your own and others) to continually improve care/practice.

A healthcare professional should not undertake a particular practice because:

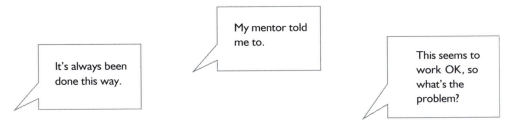

Figure 0.1 Reasons for a particular practice?

Decisions, care and treatment should be based on the best available evidence.

A multitude of definitions for evidence-based practice exist, spanning healthcare, but most offer the same insights. In the context of social care and education, the Department for Education offers the following explanation:

> Evidence based practice is a combination of practitioner expertise and knowledge of the best external research, and evaluation based evidence. It involves a careful, clear and thoughtful use of up-to-date evidence when making decisions about how to work.
>
> (Department for Education, 2012)

Referring to NHS workers, from GPs to Operating Department Practitioners to Podiatrists, NHS Wales explains evidence-based practice as:

> a conscientious, explicit, and judicious use of current best evidence in making decisions about the care of individual patients. Evidence based practice seeks to assess the quality of evidence of the risks and benefits of treatments (including the lack of treatment) that may have a direct impact on clinical decisions made by NHS professionals and patient care.
>
> (Health in Wales, 2010)

Clearly, critical skills are required for this. It is necessary to consider the evidence on which practice is based and then, when relevant, apply it to your real life work. For this to happen, you need the skills to locate relevant research, to evaluate it and then to take what is of value and incorporate it into your practice. It is also important that you can understand and question the evidence base underpinning current guidelines. Do these stand up to scrutiny or has recent research and developments rendered them obsolete, for example?

How to use this book

This short book seeks to provide you with advice and activities to help develop these critical skills. You have a million other things demanding your attention (placements, essays, dissertations, part-time jobs, families …) so you are unlikely to have the space or energy to devote a huge amount of time to a study skills book. The idea behind this text is to give you a crash course in critical thinking – practical suggestions and examples that you can apply to every aspect of your degree. It shouldn't take too long. You don't have to put off reading your texts and journal papers to make space for this. Read it alongside or whilst you are working on an assessment. Hopefully, you'll start to see a change in your approach as you progress through the book.

That's the thing about critical thinking; it isn't about following a set of procedures or learning something by rote. It is about changing your attitude towards knowledge and evidence, thinking differently. Spending a little time now getting to grips with critical skills is a worthwhile investment.

The book starts by asking you to think about your current critical abilities. Trust me, you will have them. You've maybe just not recognised them yet or realised that they can be applied to academic and professional life. Each chapter then considers a different aspect of critical thinking in healthcare programmes: critical selection and reading of materials, building an argument and writing, and becoming critical in reflection.

- Chapter 1 – Taking a critical approach in everyday life: your current critical abilities and how you use them to keep your money, livelihood and sanity in the twenty-first-century Western world.
- Chapter 2 – Taking a critical approach at university: definitions; examples; asking the right questions; the toddler and teenage questions technique.
- Chapter 3 – Taking a critical approach to reading: selecting, understanding and critiquing texts and research papers.
- Chapter 4 – Building a rational and credible argument: using and evaluating evidence to make conclusions and recommendations for practice.
- Chapter 5 – Taking a critical approach in assessments: demonstrating your critical skills in written work, avoiding lengthy descriptions.
- Chapter 6 – Taking a critical approach in literature reviews: finding, sorting and critically reading literature before synthesising into a coherent, well structured review.
- Chapter 7 – Taking a critical approach in dissertations: approaching longer, more autonomous tasks whilst retaining your critical skills; making the most of supervisors and learning to redraft.
- Chapter 8 – Taking a critical approach in reflection and reflective assessments: using the toddler and teenage questions technique in reflection; demonstrating critical reflection in written work.

By the end of this book:

- You will recognise your existing ability as a critical thinker.
- You will be able to spot logical flaws and inconsistencies in arguments.
- You will learn to consider health issues from multiple perspectives, weighing up the strengths and weaknesses of a case.
- You will be able to build a convincing argument in assessments.
- You will develop a range of critical skills for successful study and healthcare practice.

References

Department for Education (2012) *Evidence based practice. Children and Young People.* http://www.education.gov.uk/childrenandyoungpeople/families/b00203759/evidence-based-practice as at 23 January 2014.

Health in Wales (2010) *Evidence Base.* http://www.wales.nhs.uk/ourservices/evidencebase as at 23 January 2014.

Chapter 1

Taking a critical approach in everyday life

Overview of chapter

This chapter should help you consider the critical thinking skills you already have, as well as clarifying where you require further development. Beginning with an audit of your current abilities, it will focus on how you have used critical skills in your everyday life. Finally, it will demonstrate how you can use popular issues and the media to begin honing your skills and your ability to identify flaws and logical problems.

Learning outcomes

By the end of this chapter, you should be able to:

* assess your current critical thinking skills;
* recognise ways in which you use critical thinking in your everyday life;
* notice logical problems in popular issues and debates.

Rating your current abilities

How do you rate yourself as a critical thinker? Have you ever thought about it before? Do you consider yourself to be rational? Do you tend to win arguments or debates? Can you convince others of the correctness of your point of view?

Presumably, since you are reading this book, it is something you are aware of and hoping to develop. But why is that?

* Because you feel you already have some of the skills but you would like to refine and improve them?
* Because your lecturers continually emphasise the importance of taking a critical approach?
* Because it is regularly mentioned in the feedback you receive?
* Because you don't really understand what people are talking about when they suggest the need to be critical?

Please do not worry if you have the latter motive – you are unclear exactly what criticality is and how to demonstrate it. This is very common, mainly because it is extremely difficult to define, even for lecturers. Often, people are able to determine whether a piece of writing is critical or not, but find it much more difficult to explain why it is critical, what it is doing that takes it beyond mere description. In the next chapter, we will examine exactly what is meant by critical thinking in academic work.

Maybe none of these reasons resonates with you or sums up why you have picked up this book. It is important to reflect upon why you have chosen to develop your critical skills, however. The more honest and detailed your reasoning is, the more likely you are to stay motivated and, thus, make a genuine difference to the way you approach your degree work.

That 'hmmm feeling'

Before beginning a full evaluation of your critical thinking skills, it is worth noting that, in general, there is a piece of critical thinking at which we all tend to be reasonably good. Most people can sense when there is a logical flaw, inconsistency or plain error in an argument. It is almost as if something does not 'feel right'. There is a sense of unease, an inkling there is a problem, a scepticism or reluctance to accept whatever is being presented. Maybe even a gut instinct. I call that the 'hmmm feeling' – the thing that makes you stop and become uneasy. This is a good thing! Learn to recognise it and pay attention to it. Go with that gut instinct.

The most obvious place you will come across this 'hmmm feeling' is when listening to advertisements, political debates or anything else that is trying to convince you to buy/ believe/vote for something. You are also likely to have encountered it in your degree studies. Maybe you have been reluctant to accept the value of a particular model or you have finished reading a paper and felt there is definitely something wrong with it. You should take confidence from the fact that you have perceived a potential critical problem.

Unfortunately, that is the relatively easy bit. It is more challenging to understand and define what the problem actually is. You require developed critical skills to pick apart an argument, understand its structure and the evidence it is using (or failing to provide) to substantiate its points. It is only then that you can fully evaluate it, write about its flaws in an assessment, potentially dismiss it or, perhaps, offer a counterargument. This book is designed to help you reach this second, more advanced stage.

From now on, start to notice when you have that 'hmmm feeling' and, what's more, begin to question what is causing it.

Activity: evaluating your critical skills

Use the following table to reflect on your current critical thinking skills. You are likely to be stronger in some areas than others. What do you most need to develop? Can you think of examples when you have demonstrated this element of critical thinking in the past? Can you think of a way of working on it? Later chapters of this book will provide you with insights, activities and advice on these different aspects of critical thinking but you may well be able to devise supplementary ways of improving.

Critical skills in everyday life

Even if you feel that you are not particularly experienced in using critical skills in your academic work, you will have made plenty of use of them in the rest of your life (the part that isn't all placements, assessments and tutorials). How many times have you snorted

Table 1.1 Evaluation of current critical skills

Critical skill/ability	Current self-rating (1 = weak, 5 = strong)	Evidence of use	Plan for development
Can you recognise when there is a flaw in someone else's argument (that 'hmmm feeling')?		I now read the small print in adverts and evaluate the research on which they make claims	
Can you break that argument down and explain why it is flawed?			
Can you evaluate different kinds of research (experimental, qualitative etc.)?			Attend additional workshops at university on research methods
Do you have a method or set of questions/ criteria you use to ensure you take a critical approach to everything you read?			
Can you structure an argument so that you lead your reader through the points in a logical order?			
Do you actually say something within your assessments (rather than simply describing the issues)?			
Can you recognise when you should provide evidence to substantiate your point (data, reference to a paper …) and when you can convince your reader by the logic of your argument alone?			
Do you consciously demonstrate critical thinking in your assessments?			
Can you undertake reflective tasks critically – deeply questioning your actions, emotions, preconceptions and plans for the future?			

derisively at a television programme or ruined your mother's enjoyment of said show by loudly proclaiming 'as if!' (sorry mothers, but we do seem to get to a certain age and insist on watching the absolute worst *Silent Victims' Unit: Peterborough* type programming)?

Reading between the lines

Most of us take a critical approach in life. We don't believe every headline we read. We are aware that these sensational headings often have very little to do with the rest of the story. We know that 'exclusives' in weekly magazines tend to be anything but, that quotes from the 'friends of' or 'sources close to' a celebrity are likely to be entirely fictitious. We might still enjoy reading the articles and buying into the narrative. Nevertheless, for the majority of us, we can see that the purpose of the magazine is to sell copies rather than to fastidiously document the truth. In these circumstances, you have considered the motives of the people involved, read between the lines perhaps. If you are sceptical that 'celebrity x' is 'desperately unhappy, alone and putting on weight again' that is because you have made a critical analysis of the evidence and found it insufficiently convincing – the sad photograph and quotes from 'friends' are not enough.

Selecting from results

Many people look cautiously at the results produced by a search engine rather than simply choosing the link at the top of the page or the one highlighted in a different colour. Again, critical skills are informing those decisions. You are likely to be evaluating the information you have – the website address, name, brief text. You will be drawing on previous experience – reputations of the websites and companies, knowledge of the subject area. You are hopefully looking beneath the surface and questioning why the results are delivered in that particular order – becoming aware that sponsored links have paid to be highlighted in search results, knowing that websites manipulate metadata so they appear high up any list of results. All of these evaluations inform your decision on which link to click.

Evaluating reviews

Consider the last time you used a review site or simply read the reviews of a product whilst shopping online. You probably don't accept every review of a hotel posted on a travel site as entirely honest or balanced. You are unlikely to decide that each comment has equal credibility. It is worth thinking about how you arrive at these conclusions – poor spelling, overly enthusiastic praise or ridiculously aggressive criticism. Sometimes, it seems that the person writing the review has completely different expectations from you (I once decided to dismiss one of the reviews written about a hotel I was thinking of visiting. The complaint was that it was far too hot by the pool in Turkey, in August! I decided it was not fair to expect the hotel owners to adjust the climate according to visitors' requirements and thus ignored that particular review). There are well-known cases of manufacturers posing as customers to extol the virtues of their products. Or, conversely, of competitors attempting to damage reputations by posting unfavourable reviews.

With each of these everyday activities we question and consider different perspectives. We wonder what the person's motives might be, what additional information we need to evaluate something or make a fully informed decision.

Alesia and Angus have recently bought their first house. It was a big decision and one they put a lot of thought in to. There were many things to consider and lots of questions to ask:

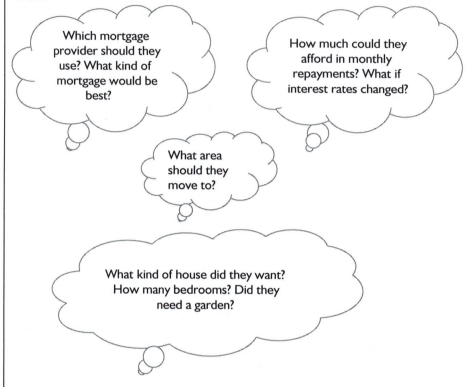

They had to utilise a range of resources when making their decision:

- Advice and information from mortgage brokers
- Advice and information from estate agents
- House schedules, home reports, home surveys

They weighed up the alternatives, evaluated the evidence, and considered the motives and reliability of those providing them with information.

Only then did they make their decision.

This process involved a host of critical thinking skills. It probably did not feel like a particularly academic or theoretical process, because it was real life, but the skills were the same. The couple came to a conclusion based on a thorough analysis of all of the available evidence.

Figure 1.1 Example 1 – buying a house

Table 1.2 Activity – choosing your current course

Why did you choose this profession?	
Why did you choose your particular institution?	
What were your other options?	
Why did you decide against them?	
Why did you choose now rather than earlier or later in your life?	
What sources of information did you use when deciding?	
Did you conclude these sources were all of equal value?	
From whom did you seek advice?	
Whose advice did you find the most useful and why?	

Using critical skills in decision making

You will have used critical skills when making important decisions. Or, if you failed to, you will have learned to do it next time, having landed yourself with a duff purchase.

It is not only lifelong purchases and decisions that require critical skills. Think of anything where you have had a few options from which to choose and the final decision is important to you – a new phone, a car, an outfit for a special occasion. Much of the time, you will have employed critical skills in your decision making.

Spend some time reflecting on the decision to join your particular profession. How did you make this important, even life changing, choice? What sources of information did you turn to? Answer the questions in Table 1.2.

Critical thinking in the twentieth-century, Western world

So you *do* currently have critical skills. They are a necessary part of modern living. If you did not judge credibility, question motives and evaluate evidence you would not have any money, for example. You would have fallen for emails asking for your bank details so that foreign princes could divert their vast fortune from their home countries. You would have believed that you had won European lotteries you were not aware you had entered or that some long lost inheritance was on its way to you. These well-known scams are attempts to dupe you into revealing personal information, such as your bank account details, for the financial gain of the fraudster – and usually to your financial detriment. By questioning the authenticity of the claim and doubting the motives of the author, you will have employed your critical abilities.

Another reason critical thinking is essential in the modern world is because of the barrage of advertising we are subjected to everyday. We have learned to doubt claims, look for evidence, question glowing statistics, understand attempts to manipulate us. If we didn't, we would find ourselves uncontrollably purchasing products and services despite our better judgement (yes, this happens to all of us every now and again, but for the most part we can resist).

In fact, adverts tend to be a great source of logical problems, fallacies and mistakes in reasoning. They are an excellent resource to train your critical skills and we will use them as examples throughout the text. For now, simply learn to read the small print. Did that advert really make the claim that 86 per cent of women agreed the product changed their life whilst a tiny font at the bottom admitted this was 86 per cent of a sample of 23 people? If so, why would they continue to make the claim and how much credence should you give it?

Practising your critical skills

It is both possible, and useful, to continually practise and refine your critical skills. As we have seen, they are necessary in everyday life and you will have utilised them when making important decisions. So, first, it is important to become more conscious of this; notice how and why you make decisions and judgements. Second, practise. Question headlines. Seek the evidence underpinning advertising claims. Undertake specific critical thinking activities. Here are a few example exercises:

Critical thinking activity 1: categories

1. Consider a topic.

- Try music to begin with.

2. List all of the different things that you can fit under this particular topic:

- For music, you might list classical, pop, rock, folk.

3. You will have automatically sorted this list into some sort of concept or categorisation. Work out what this is.

- Musical genres in this example

4. Now think of other ways in which you could categorise this topic.

- Genre, musical instruments, decades, female artists, groups, solo artists, singers, favourites

This kind of activity allows you to practise evaluating information from different perspectives, seeing data or concepts in varying ways. These categories are all types of music, but the way that you think about them, what you would do with them and how you would sort items would change depending on what category you were using.

5. Finally, consider how complicated these categories might be –
the rules you would need to establish to sort a list of songs into
their respective categories, the exceptions, the songs that could
potentially go in several categories depending upon your perspective.

- Indie as a genre or genuinely released from an independent record label or without a label?
- Classical as a period in time or any song involving an orchestra or operatic singing?

This latter activity encourages you to think about issues from a deeper perspective. A shallow analysis might decide that a song from a musical should be in the classical category because it involved an orchestral score. A deeper, critical one might decide that, actually, it would be better placed in the pop category since it was written in the late twentieth century by a well-known producer.

Go through the five steps again but use 'films' as your topic. Now try 'countries'. Finally, try 'ill health'.

Turn to the end of this chapter for some notes on this activity.

Critical thinking activity 2: arguing from different perspectives

A good critical thinker should always know *why* they think what they do, *why* they hold their opinions. Furthermore, they should be able to justify and convince others of the correctness of that view, or at the very least persuade them there is some merit in the position. Non-critical thinkers, meanwhile, may have a 'gut reaction' to issues, rely on the opinion of others or even uphold a prejudiced view of a matter. A critical thinker and a non-critical thinker could well hold the same opinion. The former, however, would be able to explain the reasons for that opinion and the evidence to support it.

This second activity asks you to focus on your opinions and beliefs about every day topics. Then begin to question what underpins those views before, finally, attempting to understand the issues and arguments from a different perspective.

1. Consider an issue on which you have an opinion.
2. State that opinion clearly.
3. Consider the basis for it: why do you think this? Research, evidence, tradition (it's what everyone in my family thinks)? At this point you may feel the need to revise your opinion. Perhaps, it was based on instinct rather than reasoned thought.
4. Develop arguments/evidence that would allow you to defend your opinion or convince others. What would you say to someone who did not agree with you?
5. What other opinions exist on this particular issue?
6. Choose another opinion (perhaps one very different from your own) and question what arguments or evidence might underpin it. Attempt to build a convincing case in support of this contrary opinion.

This latter task is difficult to do. It may be because you discover there is no evidence to support other points of view (or even your own). It may be because it can be uncomfortable to discover facts or evidence that suggest there is a flaw in your own thinking. It allows you to pull apart arguments, however, to get beyond the opinion/

conclusion/thesis and to evaluate the supporting evidence/premise, or lack of it, underpinning that opinion.

Possible issues to consider:

- lowering of the age of consent
- the right to die
- obesity as a reason to turn down prospective foster carers
- penalties for failing to vote.

Mistakes in reasoning

People can often make logical errors in their thinking. Adverts, research papers, theories can be riddled with inconsistencies, unsubstantiated or overblown claims or illogical leaps – things that produce that 'hmmm feeling' described earlier. It is vital you learn to recognise them in both your own work and that of others. Each chapter of the book will include details and examples of some of the most common mistakes.

Appeal to authority

I am a mother so I just know that I shouldn't put my child through the pain and danger of a vaccination.

Professor Sadie Banks is an international expert on type 2 diabetes. Her new theory is bound to be correct.

In both of these examples, the argument is based on the qualifications of the person cited (the mother and the professor). There is an appeal to their authority – you should believe this argument because of who is saying it or because of the person named as proof. This distracts from the argument and is illogical – is there evidence that the process of pregnancy bestows scientific knowledge of vaccinations on mothers? Are professors infallible and, therefore, any of their theories automatically correct? When put like this, the clear answer is no.

Appeal to authority arguments occur relatively frequently within adverts and politics: you should buy a product because this famous person is telling you it is fabulous; you should not listen to the details of this person's policy because they belong to a certain political party. It is important to focus on the claim or argument made. Do not dismiss it, or accept it, simply because of the person saying it.

Practise spotting this type of mistake in reasoning in the news.

Notes on activity 1

The way you have completed the three topics will be unique to you and your imagination. Hopefully, you have been able to devise a few different ways of categorising the items you came up with for each topic. The goal is to begin to recognise the complexity of the issues, the fact that some items might belong in several categories. It is possible to entirely change the way you approach the topic and the constituent items depending upon your perspective (the conceptual category you are using). This is the beginning of critical thinking.

Films – the issues you might have thought about include genre, star/producer/writer/ director, budget, based on book/real-life, box office returns, English language, awards. Deeper considerations could include deciding to put *Aliens* in the horror rather than science fiction category or deciding that animated films are not necessarily within your children's film category.

Countries – you might have categorised by terrain, language, ethnicity, political system, gender equality, religion … Do you place Turkey in your Europe or Asia category? Are France and the UK similar because of their EU status and democratic governments or different due to language and culture?

Ill health – your initial list might include topics such as disease, smoking, early death, obesity, healthcare, hospitals. These could be categorised in many ways. Causes, kinds of patients, symptoms, treatments … To increase the complexity of your categories you could begin to add other criteria or ask more complex questions – is this a socio-economic issue? Which member of the inter-professional team should take the lead role? Should priority be given to prevention rather than treatment?

Chapter 2

Taking a critical approach at university

Overview of chapter

Having considered the critical skills you utilise in everyday life, Chapter 2 moves on to critical approaches in your academic work; how you can transfer those same skills to university. First, it will consider what lecturers mean when they ask for critical thinking, before unpicking some common misconceptions. It will then consider surface approaches to assessments and healthcare topics comparing them to deeper, more critical positions. This will allow you to recognise the difference and ensure you adopt the latter attitude in your own work.

Learning outcomes

By the end of this chapter, you should be able to:

- provide your own definition of critical thinking;
- understand and dispel some common misconceptions about critical thinking;
- apply 'questioning techniques' when considering academic issues to ensure a more critical approach.

What do they actually mean?

Critical thinking is a key aspect of learning at university. It is expected of every student as they approach graduation. Yet there is often mystery surrounding what exactly is meant by it. As a concept, it is difficult to define. It is reasonably straightforward to recognise whether a piece of work is critical or merely descriptive, but it is much trickier to be able to explain where that criticality is demonstrated or exactly what is expected from a model answer, however.

The language surrounding the issue varies considerably too. Different tutors, different disciplines, all may use slightly different expressions. If you are not careful, this can make your head spin!

But whatever the terminology, you are being asked to demonstrate the same set of skills. Even though there is no one accepted definition of the term or theoretical model of critical thinking, we do know what it involves:

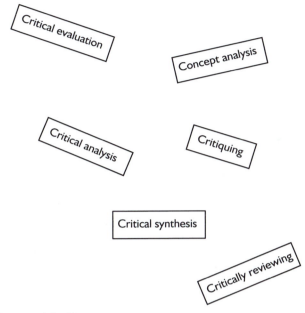

Figure 2.1 Terms for critical thinking

- weighing up an argument from many perspectives
- evaluating evidence
- challenging assumptions (your own as well as others)
- investigating the context of any work or statement
- questioning and examining everything you encounter
- thinking at a deep rather than surface level
- making logical connections between ideas and knowledge
- relating theory to practice (and vice versa).

Critical thinking is the opposite of uninformed opinion. It involves a great deal of self-awareness. You have to reflect upon your own thinking and become comfortable with the idea that there are no fixed or simple answers.

At its simplest, it is about adopting a particular stance whenever you are confronted with a new idea/fact/piece of information. Do not rush to accept or reject it. Do not, unthinkingly, file it away along with the other things you know about that subject. Instead, question it; dig a little. Wait to be persuaded of the correctness of something.

In fact, I think there are three basic steps involved in the process:

1 Get to the heart of the concept/theory/argument with which you are engaged

Make sure that you fully understand it. In earlier work, you may have only partially understood what you were discussing. You may have, not to put too fine a point on it, fudged it. If you are to critically engage with something, however, that won't do. You need to understand the ins and outs of the idea. A fool-proof way of checking that you fully understand is to ensure that you are able to explain it clearly and succinctly to someone else. Try telling someone about the concept. If they are left mystified, this might say something about your own grasp of it. If, conversely, they end up with a full understanding, this definitely means you have one too. When you find yourself in the former category, do a bit more reading around the subject or ask a tutor, lecturer or colleague for a bit of clarification.

2 Analyse and evaluate that concept

Having understood the issue, start questioning it. Where is the evidence to support this claim? Is this a logical argument? Are you convinced by it (any 'hmmm feelings')? Are there any underlying assumptions you should consider? Where does this particular concept fit with the rest of your knowledge on the broader topic and is your general thinking on this going to have to alter as a result?

It is important to recognise that no one's authority is beyond question (if you think back to *mistakes in reasoning* in the last chapter, appeal to authority was actually one of the most common errors). All papers, policies, methods and theories should be open to scrutiny. There is nothing wrong with you asking questions of some of the most accepted elements of your discipline or the most respected authorities.

3 Synthesise the concept along with others to construct your own argument

Critical thinking is more than simply evaluating evidence. That is an enormous part of it, certainly, but a great critical thinker will go beyond that, to construct an argument of their own. They will take a concept, examine it and then draw some kind of conclusion, for example. Or they might apply that concept to a slightly different scenario; show how it might be effective (or otherwise) in a practice situation. They might draw together two, three or even four ideas by exploring how they interact, or examine which is most appropriate in which circumstance.

A novel or unique argument is thus created. Often, students can become lost in the later years of their degree when they cannot find texts or journal papers on the exact topic they are examining. As you will see in the next chapter on critical reading, this is because discussion of that exact topic may not exist, certainly not in the precise context in which you are exploring it. Instead, you should find papers and sources of evidence on the different aspects of the topic, then bring them together to create your own discussion and argument.

Myths of critical thinking

A number of misconceptions exist around the issue of critical thinking.

Criticising in the everyday sense of the word

If you criticise a friend's new outfit, you will not be saying anything positive about it (depending on the circumstances, you may also lose a friend as a result). That is because in the everyday meaning of the word, criticising is negative. To criticise is to point out problems, show the flaws, the inadequacies. No one would ever shout 'stop criticising me!' in response to praise. It would only be appropriate with a barrage of negative, even hostile comments.

In academia, the university setting, however, the meaning is somewhat different. Here, criticising means evaluating. You might argue that a paper uses a really exciting methodology that appears to point towards a new direction in research. Or you might decide that the findings are particularly significant and should lead to a change in practice. These are both very positive statements. So long as you have evidence to support your claims, they will still be critical comments, however. So critical thinking is looking at the positives and the negatives.

Simply accumulating information or knowing a lot

The 'university of life' is all well and good, and those with an encyclopaedic array of facts may be useful in a pub quiz but that does not make them critical thinkers. It is not what you know, it's what you do with it that counts! Critical thinking involves deducing consequences from that information/data/knowledge. Repetition of facts is a surface skill. It is much more complex to examine a fact, consider whether it holds up to scrutiny, determine how it might be applied to other situations. It is those deeper skills you are being asked to develop.

Being argumentative

Being critical does not mean tearing things down for the sake of it. People can feel that they are being rude or argumentative when questioning concepts. This is not the case within an academic context. We expect you to do these things! And remember, you will hopefully be discerning lots of positive features, pointing out the good things and making constructive comments. It is OK to become something of a sceptic: someone who does not automatically accept things they are told but instead probes deeper, needing to hear the evidence supporting that stance first.

Following a formula

I am often asked by students if there is a set method for ensuring a critical approach, a list of questions or an exact formula. Unfortunately, it is not as straightforward as following a recipe or set of instructions. The way in which you will critically engage with a topic depends on the particular circumstances – the topic in question, the evidence you are examining, the type of assessment you are completing. So there cannot be 'eight simple steps' to guarantee criticality. You need to adopt a particular approach or attitude in everything you do. Have the confidence to ask the questions that you have decided are appropriate rather than sticking to a list that might not suit the situation.

Critical thinking in assessments

Activity: recognising demands for a critical approach within assessment questions

Look through assessment questions you have been given whilst at university (the ones you decided not to choose as well as the questions you answered) and go through past exam papers (these may well be available on your institution's virtual learning environment).

Now note down the instruction words in those questions. These are the parts of the question that tell you what to do with the specific topic. So if the question is 'discuss the significance of theory to nursing care' the instruction word is 'discuss'.

Decide which of these instruction words are asking you to approach the subject from a critical perspective.

There are notes on this activity at the end of this chapter.

Critical vs shallow approaches to assessment questions

It is often easy to be fooled by an essay question, to fail to notice that it is asking you to be critical. Unfortunately, it is nearly always possible to answer the question in a superficial, non-critical manner. You can feel you have put the work in, that you have an understanding of the topic and that you addressed the question, yet your marks will be low. Don't be fooled. By the latter stages of your degree programme, and in any further study when a registered practitioner, critical engagement is expected in pretty much any essay question, exam, reflective piece or presentation. No one is looking for the straightforward, superficial answer from you.

Consider the following examples of essay questions. For each, two possible plans have been developed.

Essay A

The Specialist Practitioner Health Visitor should prescribe vitamin D to all children under 2 years old. Discuss.

Essay plan 1

Introduction
- Role of the health visitor
- vitamin D and bone health

1. NMC Guidelines on vitamin D
- Supplement prescribed for pregnant, breastfeeding and under 2s

2. Reasons why vitamin D supplements of benefit to under 2s

3. Consequences of vitamin D deficiencies
- Rickets

4. Ways in which health visitor can encourage vitamin D uptake
- Leaflets, education
- Work with interprofessional team

5. Possible problems with excessive vitamin D levels

Conclusion
- Health visitors should prescribe vitamin D.

This essay does answer the question that has been set – should the health visitor prescribe vitamin D? Yes. All of the information is relevant and a reader would come away knowing about vitamin D deficiency and the role of the health visitor, but this would be purely factual rather than discursive. The essay also appears to be well structured, walking us through some of the issues concerning vitamin D. If this was a first-year essay, the content may well be sufficient to achieve a pass.

It is a rather shallow answer to the question, however, since there is no discussion, no consideration of the complexity of the situation. Instead, what this essay offers is a narrative approach. It tells a story. So it will almost read like a manual or textbook detailing a procedure.

The essay never asks any 'why' questions and thus it fails to take a critical approach to the subject matter. So, for example, in part 4, the essay describes ways in which the health visitor may encourage vitamin D supplement use. It doesn't ask why though:

- Why would leaflets be useful?
- What evidence is there for this?
- Are some types of leaflets more effective than others?
- Are there any weaknesses with this kind of approach?
- Do different client groups have different educational/health information needs (asylum seekers, teenagers, etc.)?

Similar questions could have been asked about the interprofessional team or even the role of the health visitor. This would have led to a much more critical piece of work.

The essay does make an attempt to demonstrate a critical approach by finding counter opinion. The final section introduces possible problems concerning high vitamin D levels. The writer presumably believes that they are demonstrating criticality by including a different perspective, by suggesting that not everyone considers the supplement a universal good. Yet this remains a surface approach, as it is an inappropriate argument, an artificial one even. There seems to be virtual consensus within the UK that vitamin D supplements are useful for young children. Any discussion of excessive intake concerns much older adults and is, therefore, not particularly relevant to the essay question.

This demonstrates the dangers of attempting to follow a critical thinking formula or to artificially introduce opposition or a counter view. In this case, it has not led to greater discussion or highlighted the complexity of the issue. There were many opportunities to include competing perspectives or consider the challenges associated with the topic. A last-minute introduction of inappropriate controversy at the end of a descriptive essay does not fulfil this function.

Essay plan 2

Introduction
- Role of the health visitor
- Vitamin D and bone health

1. Evidence-based practice
- Definitions
- Why vital for good practice and healthcare
- NMC, NICE guidelines and their evidence

2. Reasons why vitamin D supplements of benefit to under 2s
- Underlying physiology and biochemistry
- Problems relating to deficiencies

---

3. Socio-economic factors
- Correlation between deficiencies and low status groups, ethnicities? Possible explanations
- Poor uptake of supplements and possible reasons for this
- Issues of maternal health

4. Role of the health visitor and vitamin D
- Education and health promotion (link to theories of health behaviours)
- Link with midwives and GPs

5. Challenges of implementation
- Focus on prenatal or postnatal period?
- Lack of training/awareness amongst health visitors
- Limited time spent with clients
- Possible solutions

Conclusion
- Best practice suggests it is essential to prescribe vitamin D and provide education and support to encourage uptake

---

This essay takes a far more critical approach to the subject. Initially, it relates the topic to evidence-based practice, setting the scene and demonstrating the need for evidence to underpin the actions of the health visitor. This immediately marks the essay out as a considered piece of work, drawing on theory and professional practice.

The essay has something to say about the topic. It answers the question but shows that it is a far more complex issue than simple prescription. It discusses possible links between health behaviours and socio-economic factors, for example – exploring underlying explanations or causes, examining the evidence and suggesting where the role of the health visitor might mitigate some of these factors.

The second essay would certainly be one way to approach the assessment and would undoubtedly demonstrate a critical approach, discussing in depth some of the issues at the centre of the problem. It is not the only way, however. This essay question could have been answered in many ways. You may know about the topic and can think of several other formats in which to tackle it. So long as these go beyond a simple narrative or description and really get involved in debate they are likely to be just as valid.

Essay B

Are orthoses (shoe inserts) the most suitable treatment for amateur runners suffering plantar fasciitis (inflammation of the plantar fascia leading to heel pain)? The plan for this essay in Figure 2.2 indicates that a critical essay is likely to be produced; one that answers the question from a broad perspective. It begins by establishing the theoretical basis chosen to discuss the issue – evidence-based practice – as well as commenting on the challenges of such an approach.

The plan also demonstrates that orthoses are to be considered alongside possible alternatives, weighing up the supporting evidence, strengths and weaknesses of each. Importantly, each treatment is assessed from the point of view of a runner's needs rather than from a more general standpoint. The conclusion is reasoned, detailed and directly related to the question.

The second essay in Figure 2.3 is far more superficial and would not receive as high a mark as the first. There is clearly an attempt to answer the question, to research and provide information on the topics of plantar fasciitis and orthoses, but the plan suggests it is likely

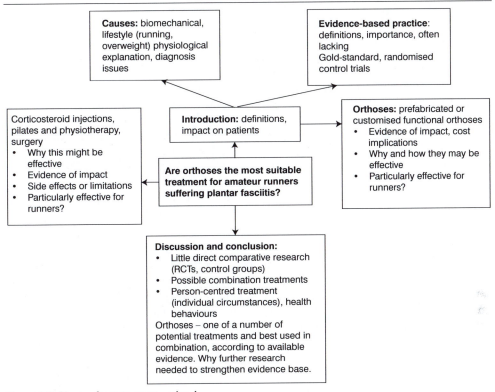

Figure 2.2 Plantar fasciitis essay – plan 1

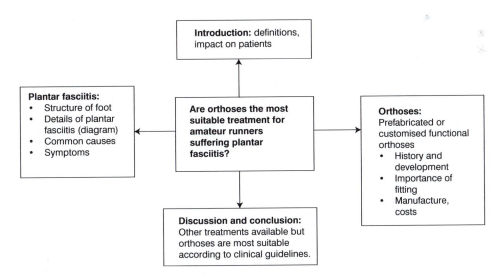

Figure 2.3 Plantar fasciitis essay – plan 2

to read more like a story than a discursive essay. There are facts and detail that perhaps lack relevance – do we need a complete history of the development of orthoses or is the research evidence investigating their effect more important, for example?

There is very brief mention of alternative treatments, but even then only within the conclusion. This means the essay is likely to have considered only one perspective and thus lacks that essential critical approach. It does not ask what alternatives might be considered. It also fails to consider why the treatment may, or may not, be effective – what is it doing, how is it working, what evidence there is to support any claims. Finally, the essay does not appear to answer the specifics of the question, that the patient/client is an amateur runner. Would they have different symptoms, expectations, behaviours and, therefore, possible treatments to a cyclist or a less active person, for example?

Asking questions

In both of the essays above, the superior plans were far more critical because they asked questions of the problem. This is a key aspect of critical thinking: probing a bit deeper; challenging and asking difficult questions.

If you take just one thing from this book, I hope it is this: ask questions, all the time, of everything. Reading a paper or listening to a lecture can potentially be very passive activities. You are letting the information/opinions/arguments/complete nonsense flow towards you. The danger is that you simply listen and accept what you have heard. This is even more likely if the person speaking is more senior than you or is a noted authority on the subject. Questions stop you taking things for granted, however. The simple act of saying 'really?' to yourself whilst listening or reading automatically engages your brain and your critical side. You won't then just accept the argument. You may, ultimately, be convinced by it, but if you have asked questions you will have made sure that there is sufficient, credible evidence underpinning the argument before coming to any kind of decision on it.

There are a couple of techniques that can help you become more of a critical questioner.

Be a toddler

Think back to toddlers you have known and loved. Remember that particularly irritating phase where the little dears are both super curious and realise how much fun it is to keep asking you questions?

It can be helpful to utilise a similar approach when tackling a new topic. Keep asking why.

- Why is this a suitable/unsuitable treatment?
- Why is it effective (what does it do, how does it work)?
- Why are they saying that?
- Why is that current policy?

Every time an argument, theoretical position or statement is made by someone, ask why. This automatically encourages you to take that critical approach – to examine the evidence and look beyond simple statements. There will be no chance of you accepting something as true just because an authority figure made the claim; you won't take a superficial perspective in an essay because you failed to see that it required you to question assumptions.

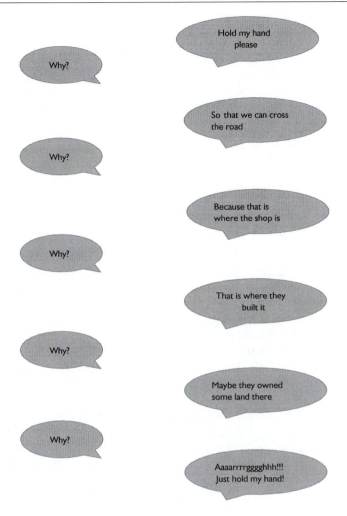

Figure 2.4 The toddler question

Be a teenager

Now think about your sulky adolescent years. Picture the sullen question associated with teenagers:

So what?

Adopting this particular attitude can also be helpful in developing a critical approach. You don't necessarily want the complete cynicism and disbelief associated with teenagers, but healthy scepticism is useful. This question also ensures you consider the wider context – why does this matter, what impact will it have, what should be done? It is all too easy to discuss a particular theory or piece of research but forget to consider its significance. Asking 'so what' does this.

Activity: avoiding the shallow answers

Asking the toddler and teenager questions leads to a critical approach with assessments. At every stage of the essay writing process (when brainstorming, researching, planning, drafting and proofreading) keep asking questions, the 'whys' and the 'so whats' in particular.

Brainstorm the following assessments. What questions would you be asking? Would any 'whys' and 'so whats' ensure you approached the topic critically?

1.   Discuss the causes of childhood obesity
2.   How important are family rooms for hospitalised infants and young children?

There are notes at the end of this chapter.

Becoming comfortable with uncertainty

Becoming critical can actually be a pretty painful process. There is no certainty, no authorities you can cling to because they are always correct. The positive of this is that it leaves you with far more autonomy and creativity. The downside is that you can have your confidence shaken and feel like you would prefer someone else to make judgements. You may feel you don't have the knowledge or tools to fully evaluate the work of experts. We'll cover this in more detail in the next chapter. The important thing to recognise is that intellectual uncertainty and doubt are OK. There are seldom black-and-white issues and straightforward answers.

For healthcare professionals, this idea is particularly unsettling. As practitioners, in many of your everyday activities, it is vital that you completely adhere to protocol. Whilst it is necessary for you to evaluate the evidence underpinning policy and best practice where appropriate, in most circumstances you must follow it to the letter. To do otherwise would be a risk to patient safety and your professional obligations. There are also matters that are fact; they simply 'are' and thus they cannot be open to critical scrutiny or interpretation. Issues of physiology, for example, cannot be debated. A white blood cell is a white blood cell: fact. But you are rarely asked to consider anything as simple as this, especially in the later years of your degree programme.

You deal in people's lives; decisions and treatments can sometimes mean the difference between life and death. It is natural, in these circumstances, that you would prefer certainties, black and white, right and wrong. Nevertheless, critical thinking and all its attending complexities and doubts, is vital to effective healthcare. I would certainly prefer to be treated by a professional who questioned, evaluated and made up their own mind rather than someone who blindly followed instructions and believed in absolute certainties in all areas of their work.

Critical thinking and your spiritual/religious beliefs

It is important to explicitly recognise your beliefs in order to become a successful critical thinker. This is necessary so that you can deconstruct or unpack those beliefs or opinions. What is the basis for them? Is there evidence to support this? Does such reflection change your mind? For some issues, this process will revise your opinions. You might discover that your previous beliefs were based on tradition or long-held assumptions that actually do not hold up to scrutiny.

For other beliefs, however, you will not change your mind, either because you feel you have sufficient evidence to substantiate them or because it would be inappropriate to expect such scrutiny of their foundations. Religious or spiritual beliefs fall into this category. They are qualitatively different from other kinds of statements or arguments. For many, a major part of religion is faith – belief without evidence. So, of course you cannot build a logical, evidence-based case in support of it. There is no proof that Jesus walked on water or fed 5,000 people with five loaves and two fishes. There is no evidence for the existence of God, but that is beside the point. Religious people have faith that this is so. They believe in it regardless of evidence.

If you do not follow a particular religion, you probably still have spiritual or ethical beliefs that are sacred to you, for which you do not require proof – the sanctity of marriage perhaps, that animals have souls. Again, these should be put in a separate category since they cannot and should not be subject to critical scrutiny.

These beliefs have no place within academic work, however, so it should not be difficult to acknowledge them and set them aside within an academic context. You might discuss religion when referring to patients' rights and needs, or you might want to examine your reaction to something with reference to your beliefs in a reflective piece but anything else would be inappropriate. For example, perhaps you are writing an essay that involves discussion of blood transfusion. The fact that some Jehovah's Witnesses believe that transfusions are forbidden by their religion might be relevant for inclusion. It would allow for strong critical discussion on rights, consent, person-centred care and alternative treatment options. Your particular feelings on this belief would be irrelevant, however. You have every right to hold those beliefs and attitudes but they should have no influence on your discussion of it within an academic context.

Mistakes in reasoning

Ad hominem *arguments*

> Smith works for the NHS so he would insist that more resources are needed in primary care trusts.

> You should not listen to Thomson's views on university funding. He has a conviction for fraud.

In the first example, you are being asked to reject Smith's argument for greater investment not because it is flawed but because of who he is. This is attacking the person rather than what they are actually saying. Maybe his argument is weak, maybe it is self-interested but you would have to consider both the claim and the evidence underpinning it to know that. Again, with the second example, is a criminal conviction relevant to Thomson's argument? Probably not. In any case, the content of his claim should still be evaluated.

Notes on activity: recognising demands for a critical approach within questions

Some of the words you are likely to have found:

Describe, define, outline, evaluate, consider, discuss, examine, debate.

Sometimes there are phrases such as 'To what extent is …?' 'Which … is the most relevant/significant?', Do you agree that …'

Are these instructions asking you to be critical?

Describe, define and outline are the only words that are not explicitly calling for criticality. Instead, they ask for a narration of the topic, a description of a particular thing. Even with these kind of questions, however, where time and word limit allows, you can always significantly improve your marks by going that bit further: defining the issue and then going on to discuss it in more detail, drawing your reader's attention to the complexities and different perspectives surrounding the matter.

All of the other instruction words are specifically demanding a critical approach. 'Discuss' means provide an overview of the competing aspects of the topic, examine the evidence supporting them and come to a reasoned conclusion. 'Evaluate', 'consider', 'examine' are the same. It would not be sufficient to simply describe theories a, b and c.

The other kinds of questions you find in assessment guidelines and exam papers also require critical engagement. 'To what extent do you agree …?' means consider the case for x, consider the case against it, consider alternatives and then draw a believable conclusion from all of that.

Where you have been asked a specific question like that above, it is imperative you actually answer it. It will not be a simple yes/no answer (or it should not be if you have read around the topic and critically engaged with it) but it is still possible to show that you have reached a definite conclusion:

Question – *Is …. of value in the assessment stage?*

Concluding paragraph – *In certain practice situations such as x and y, the assessment tool is of significant value because … In other contexts, like those involving client group z, it is of limited use due to….*

Activity: avoiding the shallow answers

1. Discuss the causes of childhood obesity
    *   Some initial questions. You may have come up with many others, of equal validity.
    *   What are the causes? Lack of exercise, diet, education, processed food, sedentary leisure pursuits, genetic factors?
    *   Lack of exercise: why does this cause obesity? Evidence? BMI (body mass index), fewer outdoor spaces (why) link to socio-economic cultural factors (why). So what? What impact does lack of exercise have? Why should we care about childhood obesity? So what – for the child, family, society, economy?
2. How important are family rooms for hospitalised infants and young children?
    *   Are they important? Why? (quicker recovery? Maintain/develop attachment with parents – Why? Evidence?)
    *   Any challenges? Cost? Space? Pressure on parents? Impact on siblings?
    *   So what? What should be done? How much of a priority should this be (and why)?

Chapter 3

Taking a critical approach to reading

Overview of chapter

The most obvious place to begin taking a critical approach in your university work is with your reading. The best students and healthcare practitioners are critical readers, so Chapter 3 focuses on this particular skill. Beginning with less academic texts, critical questions are introduced as a way of appraising the value and credibility of sources of evidence. This same technique is then applied to research papers, graphs and other scholarly literature. The chapter considers the use of critical appraisal frameworks and provides tools to assist students in synthesising literature – bringing together the themes and findings of several, different sources.

Learning outcomes

By the end of this chapter, you should be able to:

- develop and use your own critical reading questions appropriate to the text and subject matter in question;
- understand and select appraisal tools where appropriate;
- synthesise literature from several sources to develop a creative and critical thematic analysis.

Where to start?

It can be difficult to believe that you could ever critique published research or established theories. Who are you to question these authors and how can you gain as thorough a knowledge of the subject area as they must possess? Well you do not have to be an expert on a topic to spot logical problems or inconsistencies. It is perfectly possible to discern weaknesses, and indeed strengths, within research as a relative outsider to the subject matter, and you have the right to expect convincing evidence and a coherent argument before you accept the claims of a paper. It takes a bit of practice and confidence, however.

So start small, begin taking a consciously critical approach to reading with popular press articles, adverts and even films or television programmes. There is plenty of material available, especially since the media regularly discusses healthcare and science issues.

Activity: critically reading press articles

Read through the press report (Figure 3.1) on health research and answer the questions. Remember to use your critical skills when reading. Don't simply accept assertions. Examine the evidence. Demand clarification and a logical argument.

1. What claim is the article making?

     _____

     _____

2. What is the evidence for this claim?

     _____

     _____

3. Is this convincing? Do you see any problems with it?

     _____

     _____

4. Is there any other pertinent information to consider?

     _____

     _____

5. Can you see any logical problems with the article?

     _____

     _____

6. What is your overall judgement on the article?

     _____

     _____

There are notes on these questions at the end of this chapter.

You do not have to be an expert on health research methods or the links between obesity and cultural behaviour to find flaws and problems with this article. All that is required initially is a critical approach, one that asks questions, unpicks assumptions and breaks down the argument to understand if it is logical and consistent.

Transferring to academic texts

Exactly the same approach is necessary when reading academic texts. Again, you don't need to be the world's leading expert on a topic to critique texts about it. Undertake further reading on any unfamiliar topics so you can understand the significant aspects of the argument, but don't let your limited experience stop you. You may need to read papers with many different methodologies, from many different disciplines. It isn't possible for you to have a Master's degree in each and it's pretty unlikely that anyone does. It is nevertheless essential that you take a critical approach and probe the underlying logic, possible assumptions and evidence supporting any academic stance or claim.

Often people feel that they are not qualified to critically evaluate the published work of an academic or important figure within the profession: I'm just a student and they have decades of clinical experience/research degrees/hundreds of publications. It's important to realise, however, that these figures expect such criticism (in the academic sense of the word). Within academia, this is how knowledge is advanced – by others in the field scrutinising what has been produced, spotting concerns and recommending changes or further work. Everyone is

---

Obesestenders: Watching Soaps Can Make You Fat

Scientists have discovered a link between the kind of TV programmes people watch and their size. Those who watch soaps have waists 4 cm greater in circumference than those who watch documentaries.

Dr Josie Banks and her team of researchers at Cumberland County University made this striking discovery whilst examining the viewing habits of 100 families in Copeland, England's most obese local authority. They asked participants to keep a diary of their viewing habits for 4 weeks. They then undertook complete health examinations of the families, measuring their BMIs, weight, waist circumference and lung capacity. Those people who regularly watched soap operas, and said that this was their favourite type of television programme, tended to have the largest BMIs and waist sizes. In comparison, those who listed documentaries as their preferred genre were the most healthy.

Researchers were surprised by how striking the results were: 'we have produced statistically significant findings that may help us understand the link between people's viewing habits and their general health' reported Dr Banks, 'We hope this can inform public health policy and the advice we give to overweight patients'.

We were all told that watching too much television was bad for us but now we know that what you watch can also be damaging. The three main British soaps, Coronation Street, Eastenders and Emmerdale, are regularly watched by more than 10 million people each week. Could this explain the UK's current obesity epidemic?

Dr Alesia Goutcher of the Public Health Policy Institute says it is far more complex an issue than that: 'the link between television and poor health is not new. It may indicate a sedentary lifestyle for example. There are many other factors at play, however. So I would be cautious about demonising any particular kind of programming'.

It may be best to lay off the omnibus editions if you want to fit into that party outfit though.

Figure 3.1 Obesestenders: watching soaps can make you fat

considered a peer, and peers are expected to review one another. This, in fact, is the basis of the peer-review process in academic journals.

As you may know, the most reputable journals publish peer-reviewed research. The exact process may differ slightly from journal to journal but the basic principles of peer review are the same (Figure 3.2)

Not all journals are peer-reviewed before publication. This means the papers within them have not been subject to the same quality assurance process. Do they simply publish every paper sent to them? How do the editors assess the strength of the work? It is worth considering the value of journals, and the research they contain, if there is no peer review involved.

Editor selects two or more appropriate reviewers to evaluate merits of paper and suitability for publication. Reviewers are volunteers with expertise in the subject considered within the paper. In a double-blind process, both reviewer and author remain anonymous to all but the editor.

Reviewers critically appraise the paper. They consider the literature, methods, findings, etc., and comment upon strengths/weaknesses, make suggestions for improvements, relevant literature to consider, further work that may be necessary. They also make recommendations on whether the paper is of a high enough standard for publication.

Having received the reviews, the editor makes a decision on the paper and informs the authors.

1. The paper is unsuitable for publication and is to be rejected, perhaps because the subject does not fit within the journal's remit or due to poor quality research or writing.

2. The paper has potential but revisions, further research, etc., are required before it can be considered for publication. In this instance, the authors may submit a revised paper, which is reconsidered by the reviewers and editor, perhaps leading to publication.

3. The paper is of sufficiently high quality for inclusion within the journal. It will be published within a forthcoming edition.

Figure 3.2 The peer review process

The easiest way to find out if a journal does have a peer-review policy is to look on their homepage. Somewhere there will be a link or tab displaying information for prospective authors. This lets people know what will happen to their paper upon submission. Will it be sent out to review and will this be double-blind, etc.? From this page, you will be able to determine the process.

So there are two points to take from understanding the peer-review process:

1. Scrutinising or critically reading research is not being 'uppity' or getting above yourself. It is expected by the authors and is an essential element in the advancement of knowledge. You are taking part in that peer review.

2. If a journal uses a peer-review process, you can be more confident in the work that is published within it.

Does that mean, so long as you have ensured a paper has been peer-reviewed, you can read it with peace of mind, safe in the knowledge it will be credible and high quality?

The critical person would answer no. It is essential to evaluate and use your own judgement with every piece of evidence, policy, paper or text you read. It is no different for a peer-reviewed publication. That is simply more information for you to use in your evaluation. You do not know anything about the reviewers. They could be friends with the authors (some research fields are very small and those involved may all know one another and recognise a particular submission). They could be wrong in their evaluation and have allowed a major flaw to remain within a paper. They could have entirely misunderstood the argument. I am not saying that this sort of thing happens regularly, but you cannot assume that it never happens. If you are going to discuss research or use something as evidence to make your point, it must be you that has critically evaluated it, not an anonymous group of reviewers.

So what should you be reading?

We have established how important it is to read critically. But what exactly should you be reading? In the later years of a degree programme, and even earlier if you want to attain the best grades, it is essential you use an extensive range of evidence to provide a thorough picture of a topic. So you obviously need to read widely. And essentially, you can read absolutely anything. As long as you have taken a critical approach and you make clear why you are using something as evidence, it is entirely up to you what you decide to read and use within assessments. Stay away from popular sources of information since they lack credibility and often contain no analysis, unless you have a very good reason to use them. Don't simply stick to the same few sources. Read and evaluate; read and evaluate; read and evaluate …

Remember to think beyond your discipline and profession.

- Is this a topic that social work also encounters? In which case, could there be research or best practice guidelines from there that you could apply to your own field?
- Might sociology or psychology provide a theoretical framework or underlying explanation that you could use?
- Could you consult work from the economics or politics subject area to provide you with insight into socio-economic factors?
- Is this an issue where it would be pertinent to consider the protection of children and vulnerable adults? This is a concern shared across healthcare practice and into social work, education and early years activities. Any of these fields may have theories, research and practice that would merit discussion and consideration.

You can demonstrate criticality by showing how aspects from one subject area can be transferred to another as well as by defining and explaining the limits of that transferability.

Table 3.1 Examples of literature

Type of literature	Where you might find it	Why you might use it	Other things to consider
Textbooks	Easily sourced with a search of your library catalogue.	They can be a useful introduction to the topic. They are also excellent as reference material when reading research papers – you can double check a particular method or sampling strategy for example.	Do not rely on textbooks. They are merely a jumping off point for further scholarly reading or a quick encyclopaedic reference. They date quickly and, at worst, can simply be someone's opinion.
Edited textbooks	Again, the library catalogue should identify any relevant books.	The chapters are written by different people, often experts in the subject area. So you can read a variety of perspectives within the one book.	Although sometimes peer-reviewed, each contribution tends not to be subject to the same level of scrutiny as other kinds of publication. As with other printed material, they can become dated relatively quickly.
Research papers	Search databases such as CINAHL and Medline. You can also look for relevant journals then go through issues to find papers that may be of interest.	Papers are the primary source of information and evidence within the later years of your degree. They are up-to-date, highly focused and contain empirical data.	It takes a little practice and patience when you first begin reading research papers. They are densely written with specific (and initially alien) vocabulary. Remember to look up what you do not understand and try not to panic if it takes you much longer to read than other kinds of text.
Literature reviews	These are published in journals. Organisations, research institutes and charitable bodies also commission and publish them so check their websites.	A good literature review will present a synthesis of current knowledge and research on a particular topic. It is an invaluable introduction and can provide references to further literature.	These should critically evaluate and draw out the overarching themes of the papers/literature that are included within the review. Ask yourself if this is what is being presented. Unfortunately, sometimes literature reviews are little more than a description of each paper.
Opinion pieces/ editorials	Many journals publish opinion pieces by notable figures. You can also find statements and editorials by leading scholars and practitioners within the press.	Although not as valid as empirical research, the views of experts nonetheless have their place within academia. They may have significant experience and insight.	Ensure you make clear to a reader when something is an opinion. You would also need to present additional evidence to support any argument. Otherwise, you may look like you are simply accepting the views of someone more senior than you.

Type of literature	Where you might find it	Why you might use it	Other things to consider
Theoretical work	Can be found in journals and textbooks.	These may include supporting research evidence though often they can be purely abstract or speculative. They are useful in helping to explain results or behaviours.	Theoretical work should be used alongside other types of literature. Does this theory fit research findings? Does it illuminate the evidence?
Policy documents and legislation	Government or professional body websites should provide links to these.	Research can only be understood and evaluated within the wider world. This will give you the broader perspective.	Although policy and legislation do not necessarily include their own critical writing, they should still be evaluated. What evidence, if any, underpins this policy? Why was this legislation enacted?
Government reports	Governments and official organisations present and commission their own research. This can usually be found on their websites.	As with other research, critique these texts, question any assumptions, ensure you are satisfied with any conclusions drawn.	Treat government reports and research as you would any other source. It is no more trustworthy (or disreputable) than anything else. Use your critical judgement.
Non-governmental organisation (NGO) documents	Sometimes, charities and pressure groups are the only bodies to research topics (on homelessness or the impact of welfare cuts, for example). These can be found on their website and through databases and search engines.	When subject to the same level of critical scrutiny as any other research, they can be used in much the same way.	Be aware of the difference between the evidence-based statements and research NGOs publish and their more political, polemical outputs.

Critical reading questions

Whenever you start reading anything, even beforehand when you are considering whether to download a paper or skim a chapter, develop a set of reading questions. These will help you to stay focused and to remain critical: to probe and evaluate. There will be some basic questions that apply to everything. Who wrote this? When was it written? What impact does that have on its value? The remainder of the questions will be dependent upon the kind of resource you are dealing with. You would ask different things of a longitudinal ethnographic study than you would a randomised control trial, a literature review or a policy announcement, for example.

Remember to watch out for those 'hhmmm' feelings as you read. If something feels wrong, it probably is, so dig deeper and work out what the problem is. It is a good idea to have reflective questions amongst your standard ones. How do I feel about this? Am I convinced? Is there anything bothering me about it? And don't forget to continually ask the toddler and teenage questions: Why? So what? Why am I uneasy about this? What effect does that have on my overall judgement? Does a minor weakness in method mean the findings should be entirely discarded?

You will be used to having your own work scrutinised – when you submit something for assessment, your tutors read it through asking lots of questions and expecting certain minimum standards. Do the same with the texts you read; subject them to scrutiny. This isn't arrogance on your part; it's your job as a critical reader. If you are reading a formal, published research paper, you are entitled to expect a certain structure, a certain level of detail and sophistication of argument. If this is lacking, it should affect your evaluation of it.

Examples of general questions

1.   *What is the nature of this text (primary research, review of literature, meta-analysis, opinion)?* Your answer to this will inform the rest of your questions and the overall approach you take when reading and discussing the work.

2.   *Who wrote this (an organisation, individual) and what do I know about them?* Have a look at the letters after their name to find out their qualifications, see if they have referred to previous work in the reference list. If the author is an organisation (a 'corporate author') what do you know about them? Do some research to find out the nature of the group. Is it a for-profit company, a government body, a professional association or, perhaps, a charity or non-profit body? Does that change your approach to the text? It is likely to have some impact on how you evaluate the text and may lead you to ask different questions. Consider the motives of the authors or their intent in writing. Is this an attempt to sell something or to push a certain interest up the political agenda? This does not mean you should completely dismiss the content but it will obviously have an impact on your judgement.

3.   *Is the problem sufficiently explained?* Have the authors stated their case clearly? Do you know what they are investigating and why this was worthy of such examination? In other words, have they justified the fact that they have spent time on it and convinced you that you should be sufficiently interested to read it?

4.   *Is the paper well written?* You may find something convincing because it is particularly well written rather than because of the underlying logic of the argument and supporting evidence. Learn to recognise if this is happening. On the other hand, you may struggle to understand a paper, not because you have insufficient knowledge of the subject area but because it is poorly written and the argument is difficult to follow. In both of these cases, the actual argument may still be relevant and valid but you will have to separate these issues from the style of writing before you can make that decision. It may also be reasonable to comment upon an unclear style or point out that the argument lacked clarity when discussing a text.

5.   *Have ethical issues been clearly addressed?* The particular ethical issues will be dependent upon the nature of the research but, whatever the case, the authors should

make clear that they considered these issues. Have the authors demonstrated that they obtained formal ethical permission? Did they require such permission? Where submission to an ethics committee was not necessary (i.e. if the text reports on evaluation data rather than empirical research), a strong paper will explain that fact to readers.

6. *Does the text demonstrate sufficient knowledge and understanding of existing literature in the area?* Is their literature review current and thorough? If a paper does not sufficiently engage with existing literature it will not have fully made the case for its own research. You would be expected to discuss all of the relevant seminal work and show awareness of recent advances or debates in an essay, so it is reasonable to expect the same from the texts you read.

Examples of questions to ask with quantitative work

1. What is the aim of this research?
2. Is the method appropriate? Will it allow the aims to be met?
3. What kind of sampling was undertaken?
4. Was a control group or some form of comparison involved?
5. Are the results generalisable?

For a good introduction to quantitative research see Ryan, F., Coughlan, M. and Cronin, P. (2007) Step by step guide to critiquing research. Part 1: quantitative research. *British Journal of Nursing*, 16 (11): 658–663. This paper is written for nursing professionals but is useful for anyone no matter the healthcare discipline.

Examples of questions to ask with qualitative work

1. What is the aim of this research?
2. Is the method appropriate? Will it allow the aims to be met?
3. How was the analysis conducted?
4. Were themes validated in some way (verifying with participants, for example)?
5. Do the researchers discuss their own suppositions?

For a good introduction to qualitative research see Ryan, F., Coughlan, M. and Cronin, P. (2007) Step by step guide to critiquing research. Part 2: qualitative research. *British Journal of Nursing*, 16 (12): 738–744.

Examples of questions to ask when reading statistics

1. *Has everything been appropriately explained?* You may have to go and find more information to properly understand the tests used, but the authors should explain what statistical analysis they have undertaken and why.
2. *Has the appropriate statistical test been used?* For example, are they using a parametric test when their data are ordinal or categorical (find an introductory statistics textbook you like to develop a basic understanding of these concepts. There are lots aimed specifically at healthcare professionals. It is a good investment as you are likely to turn to it for reference whenever reading research papers).

3.   *What statistical relationship(s) does the research aim to find?*
4.   *If there are significant differences, what are the effect sizes? How do these impact upon the strength of the researcher's claims?*
5.   *Do the results of statistical tests support the researcher's interpretation of the data?* Is a claim being made about causation on the basis of a correlational study? Does the author's interpretation of the data depend upon a null result?
6.   *Does the statistical analysis add anything to the paper?*

Critically reading graphs

Many research papers contain graphs – graphical representations of findings or analysis. They can be descriptive summaries of data – another way of reporting results – or present tests of hypotheses, demonstrating that initial predictions were met or otherwise. As with every other aspect of a paper, it is necessary to read graphs critically. Ask questions of them; scrutinise their relevance within the overall paper, the labelling of their axes, the scale employed and so on. Again, the toddler and teenage questions are useful. Why – why present the information in this format? So what – does the graph add anything of value to the paper (or does it merely fill up space)?

It may not be immediately apparent what the graph means. A casual glance is unlikely to deconstruct it for you. So take your time. Read it carefully, making sure you know what it is attempting to demonstrate and evaluate whether this is achieved. A well-constructed graph should be an integral element of the author's argument and not just a visually attractive addition. So it requires the same level of reading.

As with other elements of research papers, it may be necessary to turn to further sources of information for explanation or wider context. Do other papers present their results or analysis in this manner? If not, why not? Do you need to consult a research methods textbook to understand the way in which the data are presented or for any definitions (what do error bars plot and what function is fitted to the data, for example?).

Here are some example graphs that demonstrate the kind of issues you should be considering when reading critically.

Graph A: the bar chart

The graph in Figure 3.4 is a bar chart depicting the average number of days research participants spent in hospital following one of two treatments. The nature of the treatment differential is irrelevant in this case (it could be one of two surgical procedures or different drug regimes, for example). The fact that one bar is longer than the other shows that there are differential rates of hospitalisation following treatment. The treatment represented by the longer bar is associated with lengthier stays in hospital. The difference between the rates appears substantial, which may lead you to conclude that treatment A is preferable.

A critical reader should note, however, that the y axis starts at 2.5 days rather than 0, which might be a more logical place. Starting an axis away from 0 can be a way of over-emphasising differences between results. If it began at 0, both bars would be longer, perhaps visibly diminishing your perception of the difference. Equally, it would be possible to visually minimise difference by extending the axis to 14 days; both would appear very small in these circumstances. So, always consider why the author has chosen the values

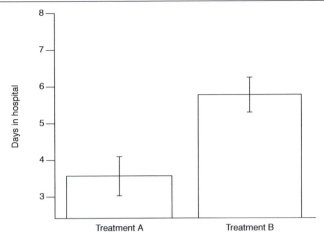

Figure 3.3 Graph A: the bar chart

and means of presentation they have. Is it to present the data in as fair and understandable a way as possible or is to show the data in a manner favourable to their argument?

In this case, although the graph begins away from 0, it does feature error bars. These show the variability of the data – small error bars indicate that differences between conditions are unlikely to be due to chance. The inclusion of such bars are an attempt by the author to be as transparent as possible with the results. So, a critical reader could reasonably decide that, in overall judgement, the graph is a fair representation and there is a difference between treatments. They may wish to mention the issue of the axis, however.

Graph B: the scatter plot

The graph in Figure 3.4 is a scatter plot that depicts the relationship between body mass index (BMI) and systolic blood pressure. You would not necessarily be expected to be an

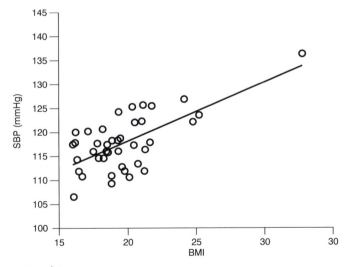

Figure 3.4 The scatter plot

expert in this kind of graph. You might never have encountered one before. If it features in a paper you are reading, however, it may be necessary to turn to a further source of information to ensure you can understand things fully.

In this graph, each point represents the BMI and associated pressure reading for an individual. The best way to read it is to look for a relationship between the two variables. If there is a relationship, you should see a pattern in the distribution of the marks. For example, if higher BMI was significantly associated with higher blood pressure this could be seen in the dots seeming to gather around a line going upwards and to the right.

The authors have included just such a line, ostensibly to show the best fit, to highlight that relationship for you. The critical reader needs to be convinced that the best fitting line is a fair reflection of the data. If you look closely at the points on the graph, you will notice that the majority are clustered around lower BMIs, with only one outlying point. Without this single point, the best fitting line could be very different. By including the line, the authors are implying a relationship in the data, i.e. the higher the BMI, the higher the blood pressure. The data is not strong enough, as displayed in this graph, to make such an argument though.

Graph C: the diet line graph

The graph in Figure 3.5 presents weekly weight loss for participants undertaking two different diets. It is important to note that points represent different rates of weight loss. Only those above 0 would indicate weight gain. The way in which data has been displayed within this graph makes it difficult to determine which group of participants lost the most weight overall, which is something a reader would surely wish to know. Such an omission appears odd. The graph does allow you to see which diet had the most immediate impact, and which maintained a steadier rate of weight loss. Perhaps this was the point the authors were trying to make. If not, one should question why they presented the data in the way that they did.

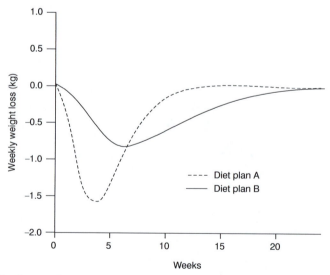

Figure 3.5 The diet line graph

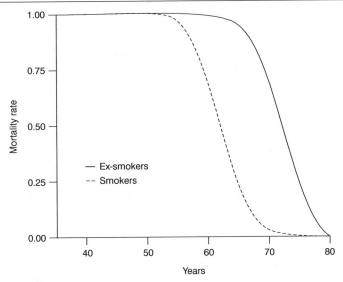

Figure 3.6 The mortality line graph

Graph D: the mortality line graph

The graph in Figure 3.6 is a fair representation of the data but it is nevertheless vital to read it carefully and critically. It is easy to misinterpret the results. It shows the mortality rate for age-matched groups of smokers and ex-smokers. The mortality rate is the proportion of each group surviving at each age represented along the x axis. Obviously, as age increases, the mortality rate drops to 0 eventually (for all of us!).

With these results, it appears to drop to 0 sooner for smokers than for those who gave up the habit. This is shown in the mortality curve appearing further to the left with the former group. A reasonable, critical conclusion for a reader to take from this graph is that the results suggest smokers die in greater numbers at younger ages than ex-smokers. An uncritical reader of the graph might surmise that the differences between the two lines mean that the ex-smokers in this research uniformly lived ten years longer than those who continued to smoke, which is not the case. Nor is it logical or coherent to infer that people can extend their life for an additional ten years by quitting smoking.

Reading research papers

If you think back to Chapter 2, you will remember that I argued there were three important steps in taking a critical approach to academic work:

1. Get to the heart of the concept
2. Analyse and evaluate the concept
3. Synthesise that concept along with others to construct your own argument.

You undertake steps 1 and 2 at the reading stage. Step 1 is essential before you can apply critical questions and evaluate what you are reading; you cannot skip or rush this stage because it is not possible to evaluate something unless you fully understand it. This means that reading papers is likely to be a time-consuming, intensive process, especially at the beginning when you are still becoming familiar with the dense vocabulary, writing style and research methods employed. It is almost akin to learning a new language. So take your time and accept that this is challenging.

I have worked with lots of students who have suddenly lost all confidence in their academic abilities. Often, they have thrived in the early years of their degree and fully engaged with textbooks, lectures and websites. It is only when they get to a more advanced stage, and it becomes necessary to read more research papers, that they experience something of a wobble. It is easy to become worried and to doubt your abilities when faced with a new challenge. It is important to remember that it is new though, so don't expect too much of yourself at first.

Research papers are written in a completely different style to other resources. They are extremely dense and often involve an entirely new vocabulary. Your reading pace is likely to be much slower than with the kind of texts you have used previously. This does not mean you won't speed up, or that you won't be able to understand the content. Have faith and patience with yourself. If you are honest, the textbooks and policy documents you now find straightforward to read, were probably just as difficult for you at the very beginning of your course. In time, you will get used to research papers.

You do not need to have complete knowledge of every aspect of the paper in question, every statistical test used and every theoretician cited. You do need to be comfortable with the general points made though. There cannot be sections that you simply brush over because it was incomprehensible to you. Don't panic if things seem to be really unclear at first. Spend a bit of time locating some reference books or websites that you like. You can turn to these to help you decode the papers. You will soon find that the same methods, statistical tests, etc., come up time and again and you'll need these explanations less and less.

Activity: reading a research paper

Find a research paper that is of interest to you (either your general course reading or something for a specific assessment).

1. Scan the paper – have a look through the title, abstract, introduction, graphs and conclusion; think about the author and the reference list. At this stage you are trying to get a 'feel' for the paper. Is it relevant to you? Does it cover what you thought it would? How is it structured? What are the authors claiming?
2. Read through the paper closely making notes. Ensure you understand the subject matter. This may involve you undertaking further reading, looking up references to other literature or clarifying a particular term or phrase. This part of the task is likely to take quite a bit of time, but it is well spent. You have to fully understand the content. If you are feeling somewhat overwhelmed, just take each part of the paper at a time. Most are handily broken into manageable sections – introduction, literature review, methods, results ... – read each one in turn and take notes.
3. As you are reading, determine relevant questions to ask of the paper.
4. Use those questions to critique the paper.
5. Summarise the contents of the paper and your critical analysis in a couple of paragraphs.

Sometimes, you will only be reading a paper as background. It might not be necessary to make detailed notes in these circumstances. The other elements (skimming to get a 'feel', undertaking a thorough read through, determining and asking critical questions) are essential, whatever your reason for reading. Be sure to summarise the content and your critical analysis soon after reading. That way, you will build up a handy, personalised collection of short notes for when you return to the papers. If you don't, even if you fully understood the paper when you first read it, by the time a couple of weeks or months have passed, you are likely to have forgotten the details. A few paragraphs of notes will bring everything back to you, especially if you have included your own critical analysis. If you like to print out papers, there tends to be space on the front page where you can write these notes (that is what I do). If you read them electronically, it is possible to add labels or notes.

Using frameworks or critiquing tools

There are many critical appraisal tools and frameworks available, both within textbooks and online. For some of your assessments you may be asked to use a particular tool when critiquing research. These can be helpful: ensuring you ask the correct questions and examine the evidence behind any claims. CASP (Critical Appraisal Skills Programme), for example, is a non-profit organisation that provides checklists as critical appraisal tools for reading research papers (http://www.casp-uk.net/). There are separate checklists depending upon the kind of research you are dealing with – randomised controlled trials, cohort studies, diagnostic studies, etc.

Remember not to become reliant on these tools, however. They are there to facilitate your critical thinking. They are not a replacement for it. You need to choose the particular framework, work out which questions are relevant and how your answers to them affect your overall judgement. Also, when writing about research it is important that you do not simply list your answers to any framework or appraisal tool questions. You will not be providing a full critique (and you will have produced a fairly boring piece of writing) if you simply answer question after question, in order, without undertaking some deeper thinking.

Sticking to the framework too rigidly

The paper is written by Jean Jacques, a registered mental health nurse with a master's in advanced research practice. She currently works at West Lanark Hospital and the University of Cumbernauld, thus suggesting both clinical and theoretical knowledge of the subject matter. Her specific role at these institutions is not known. If the research was conducted in the hospital in which she works, there might be issues with confidentiality or participants feeling unable to decline to take part.

The journal is the *British Journal of Community Mental Health Nursing Research* which is published quarterly in electronic and print versions. This is a peer-reviewed publication that uses a double-blind process. The paper was initially submitted in April 2012 and was deemed ready for publication in January 2013. It was officially published in May 2013.

The research utilised questionnaires to investigate the reasons why people failed to attend appointments. This appears to be a reasonable method to gather the views of a large …

Ethical permission was obtained from the university ethics committee. Anonymity was assured to all participants and they were given the opportunity to withdraw from the study at any time …

The sampling …

The problem with the piece of writing above is that it follows a critical reading framework too closely. It ends up appearing formulaic. It lacks insight or critical discussion and contains too many, often irrelevant, details. Do we need to know how many issues the journal publishes annually? Probably not. The order in which the paper is discussed seems to be the order taken from the framework. But is that the most relevant way to tackle that particular piece of research? Perhaps it would make more sense to comment upon the questionnaire method and sampling strategy at the same time.

Frameworks are there to provoke critical engagement, to assist you in asking the right questions and knowing what to look for with different kinds of research. They do not provide a ready-made template for critical reading, however. In fact, if you use them without truly engaging, you are likely to produce an extremely descriptive piece of work, much like the example above. Frameworks must themselves be used in a critical manner.

Tools for synthesising literature

Returning to the three stages of critical thinking and reading, having found, understood and critically read something, it is necessary to synthesise that evidence/concept/finding/ theory alongside others and thus construct your own argument. To do otherwise, is to simply regurgitate the content of a series of papers without considering how they fit together or the broader context.

As long as you are thinking and reading critically you will naturally begin to consider how the different texts fit together, how discrepancies between findings might be explained or which theory is the most appropriate for those circumstances. There are also tools you can use to help with this synthesis.

The simplest tool is a straightforward grid that you complete as you read different texts. Whilst extremely basic, this can be a powerful way to build up understanding of a topic, discern significant issues and themes, and comprehend the ways in which different arguments or perspectives fit together, or don't. When reading, make sure you have a grid nearby. Note themes, points, important factors as they emerge from your reading. As you add in more literature, you will naturally determine the points of overlap, commonality and dispute or debate. Instead of notes on three or four papers in isolation, you will have read and taken notes from them in relation to each other. This is inevitably a wider perspective, one that includes competing points of view and the broader context – all of which demonstrates critical engagement (Table 3.2).

If the papers you are reading all involve a particular kind of research, you may find that it is helpful to make your grid more tailored. It is possible to develop a grid to record critical observations on quantitative research papers, for example. You may wish to make note of sample size, nature of the experiment, etc., as in Table 3.3

You could construct a separate table for each method, or reorder them to show your results by client group, sample size or any other factor. Depending on how you prefer to work, it may be more constructive to complete an electronic grid. That way, you can reorder things more easily, thus drawing out important themes and synthesising results.

Table 3.2 Literature review grid

Author/date	Theme 1	Theme 2	Theme 3	Theme 4	Theme 5
Mckendry, 2015					
Chirita, 2012					

Table 3.3 Quantitative research literature grid

Author/date	Research design	Sample size	Findings	Strengths	Weaknesses	Practice implications
Mckendry, 2015	RCT	85	6 month programme increased memory recall significantly more than in control group ($p<0.05$)	Follow up Low attrition	Reliability of memory measure No explanation of why it was effective	Benefits to clients and potential savings in longer term care may outweigh costs of programme
Chirita, 2012	Cohort study	1050	Significant correlation between involvement in cognitively engaged activity and recall ability	High attrition	No explanation of why it was effective	
Sadie, 2014	RCT	93	3 month programme increased memory recall significantly more than in control group ($p<0.05$) though no longer true in follow up 6 mths later	Follow up Low attrition	No explanation of why it was effective	

You can use this approach for any kind of text or research. Table 3.4 provides example notes on qualitative research.

An approach such as this is extremely linear, even rigid. This appeals to some people. I like lists, neat lines and the kind of logical order that a table involves. For others, however, this can seem far too controlling and of little use when trying to make sense of the big picture. If you are someone that prefers a more visual, looser approach you may gain more by using a tool such as a mindmap when reading and synthesising literature.

Table 3.4 Qualitative research literature grid

Author/date	Research design	Sample size	Findings	Strengths	Weaknesses	Practice implications
Martins, 2014	Analysis of blog entries	7	Feelings of isolation and guilt as debilitating as physical symptoms such as breathlessness	Included 'personal insights' from participants	Broad themes were not checked with participants	Awareness of social and emotional implications of COPD within nurse training
Blackshaw, 2012	Semi-structured interviews	12	Support groups helpful but many report isolation and loneliness		Themes were not checked with participants Interview guide was not piloted	
Damer, 2014	Semi structured interviews	6				

Instead of making notes within a grid, try creating a visual diagram. Note down themes, patterns, ideas and findings as they occur to you, then make links between them. You can also try making notes on colourful pieces of paper. Have a noticeboard or wall set aside for the purpose. Do patterns emerge if you can plot them out on a large space? If you find that you are not making progress in synthesising literature in one particular way, try sorting it by another category. This is easy with the Post-it approach – simply take your notes or bits of paper down and reorganise them. Try grouping by methods, client group or practice implications to see if that creates a more meaningful overall evaluation.

Activity: using a grid to critically read and synthesise literature

The last activity asked you to critically read a research paper. This next one asks you to critically read several papers on a similar topic. Select something that will be of benefit to your programme (perhaps something you are working on for an assessment) and find at least three papers that appear to be of interest and academic value.

Develop a review grid appropriate to the subject matter and type of research you are evaluating. Read the papers and complete the grid as you go.

- What are the common themes that emerge from your reading of several papers on the topic?
- Are there areas of broad agreement and dispute? What might explain these and what is your approach?
- Are there common areas of strength or weakness in research on this topic?

Hopefully, you will have begun to synthesise and analyse what you are reading. The tools should help you perceive a more universal context for the subject rather than reading each paper/idea or theory in isolation.

Mistakes in reasoning

Cherry picking

> Two politicians are arguing about the government's funding of the police force. The opposition politician points to a report that measures the incidence of violent crime to demonstrate that the rate has risen whilst the government has been in power. The government minister discusses another report that measures the reporting of crime to argue that the rate has fallen.

So who is correct? Well both reports are measuring different things so they are not directly comparable. Also, both people are cherry picking – they are choosing evidence to support their claims and ignoring everything that does not fit. They have begun with their conclusion and sought evidence to suit it, rather than viewing all the evidence and drawing a logical conclusion. Critical thinkers complete their research, evaluate their evidence and then make their conclusions. They also discuss all relevant research, including that which seems to dispute the argument. With the latter, they demonstrate why it is less convincing than other pieces of research or explain that it is an isolated finding in contradiction to other work.

Notes on activity: critically reading press articles

1. What claim is the article making?

That the types of television programmes people watch have an impact on their body mass index. More specifically, that there is a direct causal link between these two factors.

2. What is the evidence for this claim?

A study conducted by university researchers on 100 families. Viewing diaries were kept and health investigations were undertaken.

3. Is this convincing? Do you see any problems with it?

It is an unconvincing argument for a number of reasons:

a. There could be many other factors involved. Perhaps those who watch soaps spend far more time watching television in general. In that case, the issue may be the total amount of television watched rather than the particular programme.
b. Who are the researchers? We are not told much about them. What is their discipline, for example? Have they published their findings in a peer-reviewed publication? Does this build on earlier research? Can they explain their findings?
c. We are given too few details to make our minds up. How did the researchers analyse the television viewing diaries, for example?

d.   The newspaper's claim is very strong (that watching soaps makes you fat) and it does not have sufficient evidence to substantiate such a contentious stance.

4. Is there any other pertinent information to consider?

Within the article, another academic appears to dispute the claim. Also, the difference in waist circumference is stated as 4 cm. Is this actually a substantial difference? Does it matter, for example, that there are known links between poor health and waist size? Perhaps so, but we would need to have this explained.

5. Can you see any logical problems with the article?

There may well be other explanations for the link. For example, do those who watch documentaries actually just spend less time watching television than those who watch soaps? This, in turn, might tell you that there are other lifestyle factors of relevance. Perhaps they are more physically active and, thus, have a lower BMI.

I would be interested to know the characteristics of those who typically watched soap operas. Are there socio-economic factors involved, for example? Have the researchers been able to factor out salary, size of family, gender, etc.?

The article is claiming a causal link between these two factors – that somehow watching a particular kind of television programme directly causes a greater waist size. Why would that be? What might explain this? If there is evidence of a link between these two characteristics, it is far more likely to be a correlation. They seem to occur together but one does not necessarily cause the other. This is a valuable finding and may help us understand, and have an impact on, obesity at a population level, but it does not provide us with details on direct causation.

6. What is your overall judgement on the article?

In my critical reading of the piece, I do not think there is sufficient or credible evidence to substantiate the claims made. The research itself may be rigorous and valuable but this cannot be determined from the newspaper report. I would source the original research to find out more details and evaluate the methods, findings, discussion, etc.

Chapter 4

Building a rational and credible argument

Overview of chapter

Having undertaken critical research on a particular topic, you are expected to synthesise what you have discovered – formulate your own credible and well-supported argument rather than simply regurgitate what you have read. This chapter will discuss how you go about constructing an argument and working out your critical take on issues.

The strongest arguments hold up to scrutiny because there is sufficient quantity and quality of evidence underpinning them. A thorough understanding of how arguments are constructed is, therefore, essential if you are to ensure this is the case with your own. This skill is also helpful when evaluating the arguments of others. It allows you to deconstruct the issue and highlight any logical problems or inconsistencies. Both skills will be covered within the chapter.

Learning outcomes

By the end of this chapter, you should be able to:

- recognise the need to construct your own critical argument and appreciate how you might begin drawing upon evidence from many different places to do so;
- understand the structure of arguments;
- evaluate the strength of arguments based on their construction and determine whether the premise supports the conclusion.

What is an argument?

This sounds like a rather stupid question, but it is important to understand exactly what an argument is (and conversely, what we are not referring to). It is not the everyday use of the word. So we are not talking about a disagreement, a heated discussion between two or more people. An argument within an academic context is a claim, something the author wishes people to accept. You can think of it with a legal metaphor – the lawyer presents an argument they hope to convince the jury of (either that someone is guilty or innocent). Or take a sales perspective – the argument is the product you wish to get the customer to buy.

You will find arguments in myriad places:

- within papers and textbooks
- within lectures
- within policy documents.

Most of the time, there will be lots of arguments within the one text. So there may be a single, overarching thesis/claim/conclusion within a research paper (this is what we found and what it all means), with many other smaller ones building towards it (these are the methods we employed and the reasons for them; this is what the current literature says about the problem; this is what the data shows).

When will you construct an argument?

The simple answer is all of the time. It is necessary to make a case within your work: in presentations; essays; dissertations; in fact, in any piece of coursework or even simply within class discussions. Rather than presenting a series of statements or simply highlighting the arguments of others, you need to actually say something, make your own claim. It is one of the ways in which you can ensure you are taking a critical approach. It lifts a piece of work from description or repetition of facts into more complex evaluation and analysis.

This is a tricky thing to do, however. You may be much more comfortable talking about other peoples' ideas and arguments. It can be quite a daunting change to suddenly be expected to produce an independent analysis of a particular topic or draw together the emerging themes within the research you have found. The key is:

- First, realise that this is what is expected of you.
- Second, recognise that you are not going to be able to find one source that covers every aspect of a topic for you. You will need to bring different resources together to build your case.

Constructing arguments: an example

Imagine you are a nursing student (this won't be particularly difficult if you are, indeed, a nursing student, but you will have to try a bit harder if you are studying podiatry!). You have been asked to investigate current practice in relation to the treatment of learning disability clients with epilepsy. You find that new research brings current guidelines into question and you wish to write about this and make some recommendations for practice. How do you do it?

1. Take a critical approach to the subject.
2. Draw together different texts and sources from diverse areas (think about different disciplines, types of evidence, etc.).
3. Use the evidence to build your argument.

You will not be able to find one paper that outlines all of the points you wish to make and provides evidence to support each of your claims. Instead, you build the case from lots of different papers.

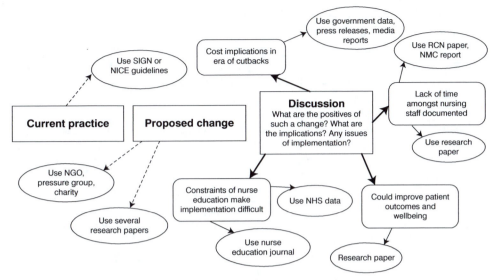

Figure 4.1 Using different resources to build your argument

Your eventual written text may look something like this:

> Whilst current guidelines insist that people with learning disabilities should have the same access to treatment for their epilepsy as anybody else (NICE, 2004; SIGN, 2003), recent research suggests this may not be happening in practice (Mulder, 2010), particularly because diagnosis can often be more difficult to achieve in this client group (Epilepsy Action, 2009). The successful treatment and management of epilepsy has been proven to have a lasting and positive impact on patient wellbeing (Brady *et al.*, 2008; Howell, 2009). This should, therefore, become one of the priorities of care of the learning disability nurse.
>
> However, in an era of scarce funding, the need for greater staff education in this area …

The composition of arguments

Arguments consist of two basic things:

1. The conclusion or thesis: this is the thing you want your audience to accept.
2. The premise or evidence: the reason(s) you provide so that your audience will believe the conclusion. You might employ evidence from published research, from statistics, from your own research or from logic.

The more premises you provide (and the better quality they are) the more likely it is that people will accept your conclusion. Your argument will be stronger. So, with the example above, it is possible to break the argument down into the conclusion and its accompanying premises:

Conclusion: the treatment and management of epilepsy should be one of the priorities of care for the learning disability nurse.

- *Premise 1:* because current guidelines stipulate that those with learning disabilities should have the same access to treatment as others.
- *Premise 2:* because this may not currently be the case (especially because diagnosis may be more challenging).
- *Premise 3:* because successful treatment and management can have such a positive impact on wellbeing.

Your task is to get your reader to believe your conclusion. So you provide premises/ evidence in support. In my opinion, sufficient evidence has been provided to make the conclusion acceptable to a critical reader. It answers lots of toddler questions (why?) and the teenager one (so what?).

It is not always obvious what the conclusion of an argument is. Sometimes, it is not stated until the end of a paragraph. It is essential that you locate it and then deconstruct the argument in order to fully evaluate it. You should break it down into its constituent parts (conclusion and premise) to clearly understand it.

Activity: deconstructing arguments to identify the underlying structure

Identify the structure of the following arguments. In other words, break them down by determining the conclusion and the premises/evidence given to support that conclusion.

1. Men are better at construction-type work because they have bigger hands. My father was able to build all of our furniture really easily. He was also good at bricklaying and plastering.
2. The studies all found that diabetes education programmes such as these were effective in improving medication compliance. The lack of control groups does need to be addressed but the results were certainly promising. Further research should be carried out to better understand their impact.
3. There is absolutely no evidence that electronic cigarettes are harmful. They should be promoted to smokers as a safe alternative to cigarettes.
4. Many people believe that sugary drinks contribute to weight gain. This is untrue, however. Research published by the American Confederation of Carbonated Refreshments in 2010 found that such drinks could help athletes maintain their physical exertion for longer.

Notes on these arguments can be found at the end of the chapter.

So why bother going to the effort of breaking down the argument into its constituent conclusions and premises? There are a great many reasons:

- to understand and critically evaluate the arguments that are presented within papers;
- to understand the underlying evidence and rationality of your own arguments;
- to help you state your arguments much more clearly;
- to explicitly express your conclusion (perhaps at the beginning) and then show how your evidence supports that.

All of which will mean that you can demonstrate critical thinking in your work.

One final reason is that it will allow you to work out whether you require a reference, published evidence, to support your argument. Most of the time, it is vital that you substantiate your claim with credible, published evidence. Sometimes, however, you make your case through logic. The premise you provide to support your conclusion is not a statistic or piece of research but rather your explanation of a problem that you have deduced from your reading. For example, your argument may be that a piece of research is flawed. How will you convince your reader of this? Well, in these circumstances would it do you much good to try to find another paper that pointed that out, even if such a thing existed? Instead, your premises/evidence involve demonstrating the issue to your reader:

- The researchers state that they are employing an action research methodology but they make no mention of the action that will emerge from their project. They do not seem to have utilised the methodology correctly and thus the research has a serious flaw.
- The aims of a paper state that they wish to examine clients' experience of post-surgical rehabilitation but the questions asked in the survey do not match those aims. Instead, they seem to ask people about their experiences during hospitalisation. So the study has a significant flaw.

In both of the examples above, it is not possible or productive for you to include a reference to support your argument. You have noticed the discrepancy between the paper's aims and methods in the second bullet point, for example. You should state your argument and provide examples and an explanation to convince your reader. This, rather than a reference, will be your premise.

Drawing arguments

For some people, it is more instinctive and meaningful to write out the conclusion and premise, like the example above. For others, it may be more helpful to draw a diagram or mindmap. The conclusion should be at the centre of your diagram with your premises moving out from there. Some premises may have sub-points, others will be entirely separate (Figure 4.2)

Figure 4.3 sketches the argument regarding the management of epilepsy with learning disability clients discussed earlier.

It can be really helpful to see an argument represented in such a manner. If nothing else, it provides visual feedback on how much evidence is being presented to substantiate a conclusion. It can also be helpful to indicate the relative strength of the differing premises by drawing some larger than others.

Whichever method works for you, ensure that you are clear what your argument is (the conclusion and the underlying evidence/premises) before you begin to write. At the planning stage, construct a diagram or write down the constituent elements of your claim.

Essays and dissertations comprise many smaller arguments or partial arguments, usually all building to one central thesis. It is important that this overall structure is conscious and explicable to you. Again, address this in the planning stage (Figure 4.4).

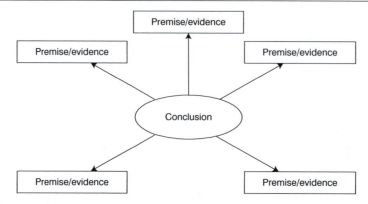

Figure 4.2 Diagram of an argument

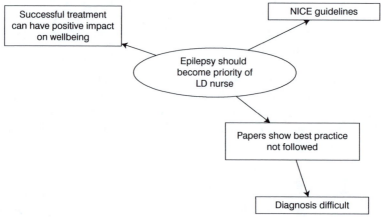

Figure 4.3 Diagram of the epilepsy argument

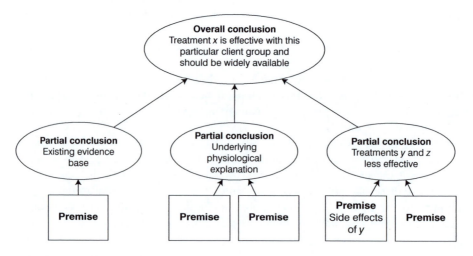

Figure 4.4 Diagram of an essay argument

Deconstructing arguments to critically evaluate them

It is possible to be pretty good at recognising when there is a problem with an argument (the 'hmmmm feeling') but it is much harder to pinpoint why. What exactly is the underlying logical flaw, the obfuscation or downright manipulation that is taking place? The truly critical thinker is able to undertake the latter task.

When you identify and understand the structure of an argument you are in a much stronger position to critically evaluate it and be able to discern and describe any flaws. You can determine whether the evidence/the premise supports the conclusion.

Activity: deconstructing arguments to critically evaluate them

Return to the arguments in the activity on page 52 and critically evaluate each of them. Do you see any problems with the arguments? Do the premises logically support the conclusions? Are there sufficient premises, and are they sufficiently credible, to persuade you to believe the conclusion?

There are notes on the arguments at the end of the chapter.

Building the 'bigger picture' argument

As discussed earlier, your assessments will rarely be made up of one simple argument. You will have many partial arguments and sub-themes. In a dissertation, for example, each chapter may have several partial arguments and one or two overarching main arguments; all of which may lead, in your final concluding chapter, to your grand thesis. If you understand how each smaller argument is constructed and make sure that, for each, your premises will convince your readers of your conclusion, you can ensure your overall structure is sound. You will also be able to check that each partial conclusion links logically to the larger ones, thus creating a plausible and critical bigger picture. Think of it like a tower block. Your final argument is the top floor but it doesn't matter how well constructed that particular level is. If the work underneath is shoddy, the whole tower will be unsound. You require each level of the tower block to be well made for the final one to be secure.

All of this means that you cannot write something (create a research poster or design a presentation) until you know what the final argument is going to look like. To be critical, you have to plan your work in advance of the writing stage. This is not a natural way of working for many people, but it is something that you need to master. You cannot just 'see where things take you' or 'read a bit, write about it, read a bit more, write a bit more'. To return to the building metaphor, you don't construct buildings without first creating a complete architectural plan.

It can be fairly daunting to begin constructing overall arguments, but that is critical thinking, and it becomes much easier with practice. If you have been critical when reading the evidence, attending lectures etc., the argument will likely have begun to form as you go along. You now need to make it explicit – to both yourself and, ultimately, to your reader. Remember the critical reading questions and reading tools that were discussed in the previous chapter. If you find a method of reading that allows you to critically analyse and synthesise what you are reading as you go along, your life will be much easier when it comes to constructing your own 'bigger picture' argument.

For example, literature review grids can be extremely helpful in pulling together the themes that emerge from several pieces of literature. You can also get a sense of the relative strength or merit of each perspective. Table 4.1 is a grid I completed whilst reading papers on the topic of spirituality in healthcare. I made notes on each paper, commenting on findings and my own analysis of any shortcomings or strengths. Slowly, parallels and differences between papers emerged.

Initially, I completed a row of the grid for each paper. With a bit of reordering, so that I was covering the same issue in the same column, I was able to write a heading for some of the columns. Finally, I could decide on the most logical order in which to discuss these headings or partial arguments.

With a bit more thought about what all of these findings and comments meant, what the overall argument should be, it would be possible to create an essay plan from the grid. It would also be useful to plot the arguments involved and to consciously discern the conclusions and premises/evidence (Figure 4.5).

Activity: diagramming your own argument

In Chapter 3, you were asked to produce a literature grid as you critically read several research papers on a similar topic. Return to the grid and devise your own argument diagram from your notes.

- By rearranging the text boxes, can you label the columns to represent the themes you would wish to discuss?
- What is your overall conclusion having read the papers?

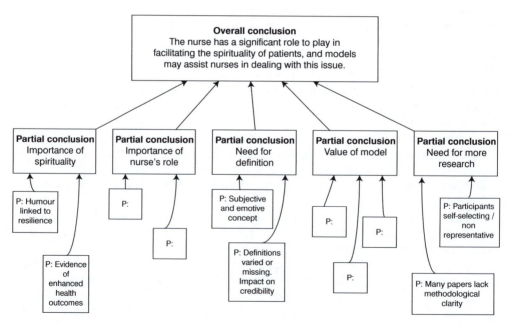

Figure 4.5 Diagram of the spirituality argument

Table 4.1 Spirituality literature review grid

Author and date	1. Importance of spirituality	2. Nurse's role		5. More research required	3. Need for definition	4. Value of model
Roberts, 2003	Importance of spirituality when dealing with life-threatening illness	Nurses' role in meeting spiritual needs	Phenomenological study – interviews with patients in recovery	Participants recruited through support and religious groups – self-selecting?	Definitions vary	
Alter, 2003	Importance of spirituality and humour when dealing with life-threatening illness	Nurses' role in meeting spiritual needs and use of humour by nurses may improve relationships with patients	Open-ended interviews lack of info on methodology Women in remission from breast cancer	Participants recruited through support groups – mainly white, middle class, all Christian		
Green, 2002	Importance of spirituality – enhances health		Analysis of literature and application of concept-indicator model		Definitions vary and require clarification	Development of model to analyse literature and allow nurses to explore spirituality in healthcare
McGonagle, 2006	Importance of spirituality – nursing needs to reflect spiritual and cultural diversity of society	An effective model may allow nurses to engage with spirituality	Grounded theory – interviews with patients, healthcare workers and public		Term is deeply subjective and much research or discussion on topic has lacked criticality	Development of model to raise awareness of structural, cultural and personal issues that may prevent advancement of spirituality within healthcare

- What are the premises/evidence you will use to support your conclusion and partial conclusions?
- Having made your conclusions and premises explicit, are they sufficiently convincing for a reader? Do they hold up to critical scrutiny?
- What other reading do you wish to conduct to enhance your argument? (Perhaps policy documents, clinical guidelines or theory would be useful in supporting your conclusions.)

Arguments are everywhere – in papers, theories, underpinning practice and within your writing. The ability to deconstruct those arguments, to break them into their constituent conclusions and supporting premises, allows you to critically evaluate them. In addition, it ensures that those arguments you personally construct are sound, logical and persuasive.

Mistakes in reasoning

Non sequitur

Dogs have four legs and bark, therefore apples are edible.

This government has a shocking record on welfare so you should vote for me.

In both of these statements, premises are presented as if they are in support of the conclusion. It is amazing how easily people can be convinced simply because they are presented with statements in a particular order or told that the two things are connected (because of this, this). But in both examples above, the premise does not provide evidence to support the conclusion. The two things have nothing to do with each other. Why does the number of dogs' legs have anything to do with apples? It doesn't. The government might be awful but that would suggest that you should not vote for them rather than providing positive evidence to vote for another party. Make sure your premise does, in fact, provide evidence to support your conclusion. Unpick the argument of others to check that this is true for them too.

Notes on activity: deconstructing arguments to identify the underlying structure

1. Conclusion: men are better than women at construction.
   - Premise: because they have bigger hands.
   - Premise: because my father was good at these kinds of activities.
2. Conclusion: there should be further research into the effectiveness of diabetes education programmes.
   - Premise: studies have found that they can lead to better medication compliance.
   - Premise: though there are some problems with this research, the results are sufficiently promising.
3. Conclusion: electronic cigarettes should be promoted as a safe alternative for smokers.
   - Premise: there is currently no evidence to suggest that they are harmful.
4. Argument: there is no link between sugary drinks and weight gain.
   - Premise: research from 2010 found that athletic performance was improved.

Activity: deconstructing arguments to critically evaluate them

1. Conclusion: men are better than women at construction
    *   Premise: because they have bigger hands.
    *   Premise: because my father was good at these kinds of activities.
    I am not persuaded by the argument. Why would bigger hands be of benefit? Arguably, for precise tasks, smaller hands would be more effective. What about automated processes that require computer rather than manual construction? Does a sample of one person (from over 3 billion men) lead to reliable conclusions? There are probably many men who are terrible at building furniture, bricklaying and plastering. Also, there is no comparison argument involving women's abilities.
2. Conclusion: there should be further research into the effectiveness of diabetes education programmes.
    *   Premise: studies have found that they can lead to better medication compliance.
        Premise: though there are some problems with this research, the results are sufficiently promising.
    This holds up to critical scrutiny. The strength of the conclusion matches the evidence. The author is not stating that these programmes should be adopted, merely that the results were promising enough to warrant further research. A stronger approach would not be tenable since there are problems with the research.
3. Conclusion: electronic cigarettes should be promoted as a safe alternative for smokers.
    *   Premise: there is currently no evidence to suggest that they are harmful.
    This argument is deeply suspicious. Just because something appears to be less harmful than another thing, does not mean that it should be promoted. Arguably the best thing a smoker can do is to give up all tobacco and nicotine products, so perhaps that is what should be advocated. Also, the fact that there is currently no evidence to suggest harm does not mean that this will remain the case. Future research may further our understanding and demonstrate harmful effects.
4. Argument: there is no link between sugary drinks and weight gain.
    *   Premise: research from 2010 found that athletic performance was improved.
    I would be concerned about the value of research conducted by such a vested interest. The confederation is likely to have considerable business concerns in the sale of sugary drinks and would not wish for them to be universally considered unhealthy. There is a huge difference between the two groups of people considered within the argument. Athletes would have very different lifestyles and needs from the general population, and those who are overweight in particular. Finally, being able to exercise for longer will not necessarily lead to weight loss (there are other factors involved, such as calorie intake for example).

Chapter 5

Taking a critical approach in assessments

Overview of chapter

Critical thinking is necessary in every aspect of your studies and your professional clinical practice. You demonstrate that critical approach in your assessments, usually through your writing. In my experience, many students are proficient critical thinkers and readers but they fail to show this criticality within their work and thus do not gain high marks. This chapter specifically addresses that issue – demonstrating critical thinking in your writing. It begins by examining the building blocks of academic writing and structure, before moving on to the features of critical writing. It then investigates how you can best demonstrate a critical approach in assessments such as exams and presentations.

Learning outcomes

By the end of this chapter, you should be able to:

- recognise what constitutes a clear academic writing style;
- understand the difference between descriptive and critical writing;
- recognise ways to demonstrate a critical approach in different types of assessments.

Academic writing – the building blocks of academic discourse

The majority of assessments you complete at university involve writing. This might be in the form of:

- essays;
- reports;
- written answers under exam conditions;
- dissertations;
- case studies;
- annotated bibliographies.

You will continue to undertake a great deal of writing once qualified – case notes, reports, academic papers, care plans, assessments for further qualifications. It is, therefore, essential that you can write in a clear and precise academic style. If you cannot write well, you will not be able to explain your critical concepts, complex understanding and original synthesis, everything that is required of healthcare students in the latter stages of their programmes.

You may feel confident in your writing but it is still worth reflecting upon. It is possible to have done well in early assessments without really getting to grips with your writing style. It is sometimes only later, as you are required to engage with more difficult concepts, discuss a wider field of evidence, or complete more lengthy assessments that an unclear style can become a major impediment.

Academic discourse (writing/discussion) is different from other forms of writing. Narrative writing, poetry or storytelling, can often be designed to evoke emotion or might allow readers to interpret meaning in several different ways. Journalistic writing may be intended to provide a brief overview or represent only one side of a discussion. Good academic writing, however, should provide as clear and precise an exposition as possible. There should be no emotional manipulation, no flowery detail, just formal vocabulary and a logical structure. A clear academic writing style makes the difference between getting your argument across to the reader or not. You can have the best ideas, have undertaken the most insightful critical analysis, but no one will recognise this unless you can detail it in a formal written style.

Consider the two examples of writing below:

> Several theories have been posited to explain the reluctance of young males to seek treatment. Reid and Mitchell (2012) have argued that a socio-cultural paradigm that emphasises independence as a male virtue plays a significant role in this phenomenon. Studies involving male interviewees appear to substantiate this view finding that many individuals regarded the seeking of health advice as something 'weak' (Goutcher, 2014; Jacques, 2011). This remains only a partial explanation, however …

> We don't really know why men don't seek health treatment as often as women do but many people have tried to come up with reasons. Could it be because they think it might stop them looking macho? Could it be because there is far more media and health promotion attention paid to women's health? Could it be that men remain unaware of the symptoms or warning signs of common male illnesses? Research has been conducted to try to find out these things and there have been some absolutely amazing results.

The first extract is written in a relatively strong academic style. The sentence structure is clear, the terminology precise and published evidence has been provided where necessary. The second extract probably has some interesting things to say on the topic but the writing style detracts from that. The manner of writing, the use of a series of questions, is inappropriate in an academic context. It is written in too informal a style (don't, we, come up with, macho) with inappropriate appeals and judgements within the language. You may think that something is 'amazing' but you should not state that. Instead, discuss why the results are unexpected and amaze your readers in that way. There is also no evidence included in the second extract. Who are the 'many people' referred to? What 'research has being conducted'?

Activity: reflecting on your writing style

Find a piece of your own academic writing (an old essay for example). Try to review the text as if you are reading it for the first time, as a reader rather than the writer of work.

- Identify three strengths in your writing style.
- Identify three weaknesses.
- Determine three specific things you can do to improve your writing in the future.

Strong academic writing

By taking a critical approach to your own writing and to all of the reading that you undertake, it is possible to discern the features of strong academic writing.

I think the following features are vital:

1. *Clarity:* Academic writing should not leave anything open to interpretation or misunderstanding. Aim to be as clear as possible. This is more important than the elegance of your writing. Hopefully you will have both but your priority is making yourself understood. Try not to be too concerned with sounding intellectual. You will demonstrate your cleverness and the complexity of your thinking through your arguments rather than through your verbosity. Try to read over your work from the perspective of your audience. Would you be able to follow this if it was your first time reading it and you did not know anything about the subject beforehand?

2. *Saying precisely what you mean:* If you want the reader to understand a particular point, make sure you spell it out to them. Do not leave them to draw their own conclusions from what you have said. State those conclusions within your work. It is then up to the reader to decide whether to accept them or not (and if you have presented sufficient, credible premises to support those conclusions, they will). To put it another way, if you think X plus Y equals Z, don't simply write X+Y and assume that everyone can work out that this must, therefore, =Z. Actually state this rather than leaving it to your reader to piece the argument together – that is not their job and they may get it wrong.

3. *Short sentences and clear paragraphs:* Consider the building blocks of your writing – the sentences and paragraphs. This will make you more aware of clarity and overall structure. In my experience, shorter sentences are often better. It is easy to lose your thread or try to put too many ideas together when writing. This is often displayed in overly long sentences. It makes it much harder for a reader to follow and important points can be lost. Again, concentrate on explaining your argument clearly rather than worrying about appearing intellectual or sufficiently 'academic'.

   You break your writing up into sections by way of paragraphs. They let the reader know that the argument is moving on. Make sure your paragraphs are of an appropriate length and consider starting a new one each time you begin a new topic or sub-topic. There is no magic size for paragraphs but they should be more than one sentence and less than an entire page. A good guide is to look at the pages of your writing simply from the perspective of your paragraphs (zoom out to see an entire page on your computer screen). Do you have lots of little paragraphs? That will make your writing look disconnected, as if you have failed to discuss the issues to any depth but have instead skipped from point to point. Conversely, perhaps you have paragraphs that cover nearly the whole page. This suggests a lack of structure, that you have not separated your work into a logical order that leads your reader through the argument.

4. *Actually having something to say:* I have had many students referred to me for writing support by their tutors. I am told that they have poor academic writing skills or that their work is impossible to understand. When I read their essays, I often agree that it is very confusing. On speaking to the student, however, it becomes clear this is not a problem concerning their ability to write (their awareness of the form and function of academic writing, of the rules of grammar and sentence construction). The issue is that they did not know what they were trying to say, or that they didn't actually have anything to say. It is only once you have completed all of your research, formulated an argument/decided how you feel about an issue, and written a plan, that you can hope to write with any confidence and clarity. Even when it comes to individual paragraphs and sentences, think, what is it that I am trying to communicate here?

    In academic work, it is never a good idea to simply start writing, with no clear idea of what you wish to say, and just see what emerges from your typing. This may produce a wonderful piece of performance poetry, but it will not lead to a well-argued, easily understood assessment. Complete your research, work out what you want to say, build your argument so that you have sufficient evidence to convince your readers, write a plan and then begin to write.

5. *Knowing what you are talking about:* Sometimes people do not know what they wish to say because they have not fully understood the topic under discussion. You cannot hope to explain something to your reader if you do not understand it yourself. In fact, as we have said before, being able to explain an idea/theory/method to someone else is the best way of proving that you understand it. So don't try to discuss things you haven't fully figured out. If it is a significant aspect of the topic, get your head around it somehow, with support from your tutors if necessary. If it isn't, and you are short of time, consider leaving it out.

    Some people worry that when they explain things in their own words, those words don't sound as fancy or intellectual as the original text. So long as you are writing in a formal style, this really doesn't matter. You will still be demonstrating understanding and writing in a clear manner. It is far better to write in a straightforward style about something you truly understand than hide your confusion behind flowery language.

Poor academic writing

As well as noticing the features of strong academic writing in the work of others and consciously incorporating it into your own, it is useful to be aware of the characteristics of poor writing. These are the ones to avoid! When proofreading, it might be worth asking yourself if you have done of any of these things.

I think there are two questions to ask yourself when writing:

1. What am I trying to say?
2. Does my reader understand what I am saying?

Table 5.1 Poor academic writing

Feature	Solution
Repetition	Lack of confidence sometimes leads people to state things several times over (in different ways). A thorough proofread should show you if this is the case. Repetition often creeps in if you have not planned correctly and so you mention the same point in several places. It can also happen if you do not have enough to say to fill the word count. Do further reading if you find this is happening. That should lead you to more discussion points.
Too many ideas pushed together	Proper planning and proofreading will prevent this. Remember, most sentences should have only one point to make. Most paragraphs should address just one topic. Think about your reader and ask yourself what you are trying to say in this particular section. If it is three or four separate points, perhaps they should be broken down into different parts.
No order to the topics under discussion	Most people's minds work quickly and in a pretty haphazard manner – thoughts occur to us seemingly at random. Your writing should not appear like that, however. It is vital that there is a logical order to your work. Start at the beginning, lay the groundwork, then take your reader slowly through all of the issues before drawing conclusions and summarising.
Description rather than analysis	Take a critical approach: draw out implications; consider alternatives (do everything that has been discussed in this book in fact!).
Clumsy punctuation (run-on sentences, incomplete sentences, underuse or overuse of commas)	Read your work aloud to yourself. It might feel weird but you will soon realise when a sentence is too long or is incomplete. It is also worth picking up a good university guide to grammar or go and speak to the learning support people at your institution. Hopefully, they'll have helpful leaflets on grammar and punctuation.
Over-reliance on certain vocabulary and phrases	Use a thesaurus (with caution). Practise writing and consciously try to extend your vocabulary. In some ways, this will happen naturally as you undertake more and more reading and become familiar with the language of your discipline. You will also develop your writing style the more you do it.
Flowery language	Some writing can look like it's had a thesaurus thrown at it (hence my advice for caution above). If you understand the discipline-specific terminology in a paper, there should not be any reason why you can't understand the rest of it. If you are having trouble, consider the writing style. Is it too flowery or over the top? Avoid it in your own work. It never helps with clarity.
Irrelevant detail	Humans like story telling. We enjoy putting in as much detail as possible – embellishing, painting a picture. That is not appropriate in academic work though. You might spend a lot of your word count on background detail or information about the author's educational history rather than fully explaining the results of their experiments. You will have a lot to say, so be sparing with detail. Is it necessary to fully understand the context or issue? If not, leave it out.
Fudging it (not fully understanding what you are discussing)	That's easy. Make sure you do understand it. Undertake further reading, try going back to simpler material or ask for support from your tutors/lecturers/mentors and your colleagues.

If you get the first sorted out before you start, when planning, you will find writing much easier and the end product will be better. If you think about the second as you read over your work, you will make sure it's clear. The best way to improve your writing is to practise and always be aware of the writing style in anything you read.

Planning written work

Alongside formal writing, good use of punctuation and a complete understanding of the topic, strong, critical assessments require thorough planning. Once you have finished your research and completed any literature grids, you should pause before beginning your first draft. Now is the time to consider what you want to say and the order in which you should say it.

If you construct a plan, you ensure you have a logical order to your writing. It prevents repetition, makes sure you answer the question that has been set and, ultimately, leads to a more coherent piece of work. It also lets you explicitly consider where and when you are going to include your critical perspective (you won't forget to discuss alternative explanations or fail to draw out the implications of any research you are discussing if it is specifically noted in your plan). I've read an awful lot of essays, and 99 times out of 100, I can tell how much time has been spent on planning based on the final product. The best work doesn't happen by accident. It has to be thought through first.

It doesn't really matter how you plan, so long as you do. In my opinion, the more detailed your plan is, the better. When I am about to write something, I'll initially brainstorm all of the issues I think I need to cover. Then I decide on the correct order for those topics (and there is a basic order for these things that will be covered below). Next, I make very rough notes or bullet points on what I want to address for each topic – the main points, models, references I am going to use. So, before I start writing, I know what each section is going to cover and what the final conclusion or argument will be.

You might prefer to construct a mindmap plan, or break things down using the word limit for that assessment (work out how many words you will write on each topic as a rough guide). Try different methods but definitely spend time planning; construct that argument, consciously include the elements that demonstrate your critical approach and think about including sufficient evidence to persuade your reader.

Structure in written work

Academic writing has a specific style, one that prioritises clarity and evidence, and uses formal language. It also has a specific structure. For academic papers, you have probably already noticed that they tend to follow a particular pattern (introduction, literature review, methods, results …). The same is true of essays. There is a basic structure that should be followed, unless you have a very good reason not to.

Signpost that structure to your reader. It is always much easier to understand something if you know what is coming up and where things are leading. So make it clear to your reader where you are in the overall argument. Make your case explicit near the beginning of the essay and follow the order you have indicated. You can also provide signposts by quickly summarising towards the end of a section and linking things back to the overall question.

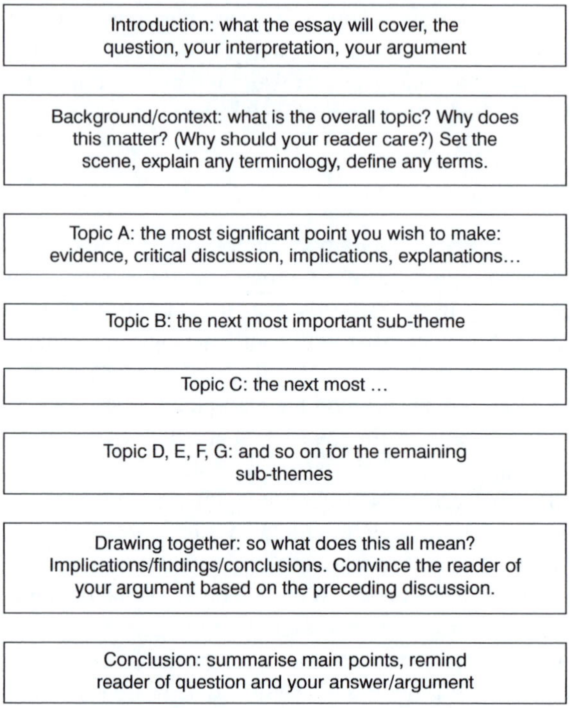

Introduction: what the essay will cover, the question, your interpretation, your argument

Background/context: what is the overall topic? Why does this matter? (Why should your reader care?) Set the scene, explain any terminology, define any terms.

Topic A: the most significant point you wish to make: evidence, critical discussion, implications, explanations…

Topic B: the next most important sub-theme

Topic C: the next most …

Topic D, E, F, G: and so on for the remaining sub-themes

Drawing together: so what does this all mean? Implications/findings/conclusions. Convince the reader of your argument based on the preceding discussion.

Conclusion: summarise main points, remind reader of question and your answer/argument

Figure 5.1 The basic structure of an essay

Features of critical writing

Having mastered the basics of academic writing, the next step is develop your critical writing skills. This involves drawing together aspects of critical thinking and reading to present a persuasive argument. Follow these tips to improve your writing:

- Introduce alternative arguments/viewpoints/evidence that appear to refute your position. Then explain why these are less convincing than your thesis.
- Draw out the implications of what you are describing and make conclusions. Do not leave anything unsaid.
- Make links with practice. What does this mean for the profession? What impact might these findings have?
- Answer the toddler and teenage questions (Why? So what? What does it mean? How significant is it?)
- Consider and discuss the strengths and weaknesses of all of the evidence you are presenting.
- Synthesise your reading. Don't simply describe one resource or piece of research after another. How do they fit together? Which papers have similar findings? What about those that disagree? What are the overall themes?

Perhaps the most important thing is to keep descriptions to a minimum. Give the details you need to explain something but avoid any extraneous detail. Quickly move on to the critical discussion. This is where the interesting stuff takes place, in the evaluation and analysis. You will obviously need to undertake some description, in the background section, for example. Make this as succinct as you possibly can, however.

Activity: recognising critical writing

Read the following extracts of writing on the topic of spirituality in healthcare and answer these questions for each piece of writing:

1. Is this an example of critical or descriptive writing?
2. What makes it critical (if it is)?
3. If it is not critical, what could be done to improve it?

There are notes on these extracts at the end of this chapter.

Extract A

There is a great deal of evidence to suggest strong links between spirituality and health. Luton and Dipsey (2008) investigated the blood pressure of religious smokers in comparison to non-religious smokers. They found that the former group were eight times less likely to have abnormal blood pressure. Another study (McLittle, 2010) investigated the experiences of 600 HIV positive patients. Those who described themselves as actively religious were less fearful of death and rated their daily standard of health as higher than other groups. Lave (2009) questioned 40 patients with bowel cancer about the role of spirituality in their life. He discovered that all but 5 of the patients considered themselves more spiritual as a result of their diagnosis. In addition, 75% of them said that they were just as concerned about their spiritual needs as they were about their health needs.

Extract B

Mitchell (2012) conducted a study examining patients' experience of humour in their care and recovery from breast cancer. Semi-structured interviews were undertaken with nine women recruited from breast cancer support groups within one geographical area in the US. The resulting data were subject to descriptive analysis to derive narrative themes. Mitchell concluded that humour was an important coping factor for patients and that nurses should use it to develop more trusting relationships with patients.

The paper provides further evidence of the importance of humour and spirituality for cancer patients. However, it fails to give a precise definition of spirituality and blurs the distinction between spirituality and religion. As Little (2009) has argued, both concepts are difficult to define and can have different meanings to different people. Such lack of clarity is problematic in a project that specifically asks patients to consider the importance of the concept. In addition, there is no discussion of ethical considerations involved in the study. It is vital that researchers (Rudolf, 2005) and nurses (NMC, 2010) gain ethical consent before conducting research yet no information is provided as to how, and indeed if, this was achieved.

As the research was undertaken in the US, there are limits to the transferability of Mitchell's conclusions and implications. The US healthcare system is very different to that of the UK (Lewis et al., 2011) with a higher proportion of private healthcare providers (Dallas, 2007) who may be in a position to place greater emphasis on the spiritual needs of patients. As a population, the US is more religious than the UK (WHO, 2013). Spirituality and humour may, therefore, be of greater concern in that country.

Extract C

There is a large body of research that suggests that patients can have improved health outcomes (Lince & Dival, 2006) and a better healthcare experience (Trupsey, 2011; Marra, 2011) if their spiritual needs are taken into consideration by nurses. For example, nurses could help patients strengthen their coping strategies or provide access to prayer facilities or spiritual professionals (Reynolds, 2006). Indeed, good practice guidelines (NICE, 2004; NANDA, 2009) emphasise the need for nurses to support patients and carers in making sense of life events.

The completion of a spiritual needs assessment should be one of the key priorities of nurses, particularly those involved with the elderly or in palliative care settings. There is evidence that nurses can often be reluctant to engage patients' in discussions of this nature (Beattie, 2007). Therefore, greater training should be given to this often under-recognised aspect of patient care.

Taking a critical approach in essays

The question

Essays are probably the most straightforward written assessment you will be asked to produce. Usually, you are given a question or statement to discuss or you have several options from which to choose. Where there is a choice, be conscious of the need for critical discussion when making your decision. Does one of the questions lend itself to such discussion more obviously than the others? Are you aware of debate or competing perspectives? This will make life much easier.

Take a bit of time unpicking or deconstructing the question before rushing headlong into your research. What *exactly* are you being asked? What are the instruction words, and are there any elements that ask you to limit your focus? For example, you may be asked to consider a treatment in relation to a specific client group. If so, you should only make reference to other groups if you can create a link or demonstrate relevance to the one you were asked about. Otherwise, you are not answering the question you were given. Think back to Chapter 2 and the essay questions and plans that were presented. It is so easy to take a superficial approach in your answer. The question will be demanding a level of criticality from you, so be sure to provide it.

Are there any assumptions within the question or task? Does it assume that intervention is automatically a good thing, for example? Is this worth pointing out or even cross-examining in detail? It may be that you have decided to take the question in a particular direction or have yourself made a number of assumptions. Make sure you make these decisions, and the reasons underlying them, visible to your reader when it comes to writing up.

Finally, this may sound obvious, but it is too often forgotten: actually answer the question you have been given. Submit the essay you were asked for, not the one you wish you had been set or the one you thought you had been given. When reading for an assessment, it is possible to become distracted. One piece of research leads you to another, and that to another, each on a slightly different topic or moving you subtly away from the main focus of your essay. It is important to keep reminding yourself of the essay question. Keep it around you and refer to it whilst reading, planning and writing. That way, you won't go off at a tangent and will, instead, be sure to write the essay that has been asked of you.

Build an argument

In order to be critical within essays, it is necessary to build an argument within your writing. This is covered in more detail in other chapters. For now, however, you need to note that it is important to actually say something about the topic within your essay. A series of statements, facts or descriptions of the various elements involved will not be enough.

You should not sit on the fence about the topic either. It is obviously necessary to provide balance, to discuss all aspects of the issue and all relevant points of view but they should not all be given equal weight. Do not leave it to your reader to decide which is the most valid. Your argument may well be 'there are a number of relevant factors' but you will need to be a little more specific than that. Which two or three factors are the most relevant and why? If there are two sides to the debate, which is the most convincing for the particular circumstances you are discussing and why? This need not be completely black and white. You do not need to totally dismiss one theory and wholly accept the other. They may both have strengths and weaknesses, and it is worth reiterating that in your conclusion. But, ultimately, you must make sure you are actually saying something; you are making some kind of evidence-based judgement.

Remember that your argument must be based upon convincing evidence. Whilst it is necessary to come to some kind of conclusion, you will need to persuade your reader of the validity of that conclusion. You will use evidence and logic to demonstrate that this is the correct answer to the question you have been set. Do not simply state your conclusion and expect it to be accepted.

Finally, when it comes to essays and building an argument, keep checking that you are taking a critical approach and that you have not fallen into the trap of description. Long sections that provide a narrative, lots of largely irrelevant detail, chunks of quotations – these are all warning signs that you are being overly descriptive. You are not really saying anything in these sections. You are simply providing facts or recounting the views of others. Only provide the details that are necessary for context and move quickly on to the critical stuff: the discussion, evaluation, synthesis and search for meaning and application.

Taking a critical approach in exams

With other kinds of assessments, it is just as important to demonstrate your critical thinking. Examinations are no exception. Plan carefully, avoid simple description and discuss the issues. This is true of both your exam preparation and the way that you answer the questions during the exam.

A critical approach to revision

Thinking critically actually helps with revision. Don't just revise the facts of a theory or clinical condition. Think about its implications, alternatives, underpinning evidence. That way, you will understand and remember a much wider array of detail than those bare facts alone, and can employ them all when it comes to the exam.

Even when memorising is necessary, remembering the correct physiological terminology or the specific order of a technique for example, it still helps to make your revision self-consciously critical. Think about why you have to learn this particular thing. If you place the facts in context, alongside your other knowledge rather than as an isolated fact, you are much more likely to remember it when it comes to the exam. All of the neighbouring information can act as a memory trigger if you are not immediately able to recall the exact details you require.

Perhaps you are revising the endocrine system. Rather than simply going through the labels over and over until you are confident you have committed them to memory, revise the system alongside the context, the other aspects of this topic that are relevant to the exam. So maybe it was part of a larger unit that also investigated diseases of the endocrine system such as diabetes mellitus or thyroid disease. Even if it wasn't, if you can make these connections, it will bring the topic alive for you, help with your revision, improve recall in the exam and remind you why the topic is important to real-life healthcare. Have you had any clinical experience of patients with these issues? What are the symptoms and prognosis? How does this relate to the underlying physiology?

Activity: the toddler and teenage questions whilst revising

Set about revising for a topic as you usually would. So you might:

- make a copy of your notes;
- create a mindmap;
- develop a set of revision notes on cards or yellow stickers;
- colour code your lecture notes;
- go through your essays with a highlighter.

Once you have been through the topic, it is time to test yourself to see how effective your revision has been. This will let you know which elements you now understand well and which require further work.

One of the best ways to test yourself and to ensure you have a critical understanding of the issues is to use the toddler and teenage questions that were introduced in the critical reading chapter. Each time you make a statement, remember a fact, answer a practice question or draft an exam essay plan, keep asking yourself 'why?' and 'so what?'. This will make you search deeper for answers, add relevant detail and include critical discussion where appropriate.

Longer exam questions

There are many kinds of exams and you are likely to encounter a mix of them during your programme. The question types will also vary, from multiple choice to missing words, short answers to longer essay-type questions. These latter questions will require the same level of critical engagement as essays. In the later years of your degree, examiners require a depth of knowledge, understanding and discussion from you. The regurgitation of factual information alone will not demonstrate this.

The tendency to simply narrate facts and description is even greater under exam conditions (you are nervous and want to fill the page really quickly) so don't fall in to the trap. Don't rush to begin writing and then simply note down whatever comes into your head in the order in which it arrives. As we have seen with essays, this does not produce a logical or well-argued answer. So, just as with essays, take a little time to plan your answer. Unpick the question to be sure you have understood it (again, given nerves it is easy to misread something) and consciously include critical discussion in your plan. Only then begin to write. This way, you will have a structure to your work, an introduction, main section and conclusion, there will be an order to the topics and you can lead your reader through the argument. Obviously, time is precious so you have to do all of this fairly quickly, but it is well worth doing.

No one expects an essay produced under exam conditions to be a polished piece of writing. You may remember an additional topic you would like to cover half way through writing so that you need to change the order, cross out sections or use symbols, such as an asterisk, to show which paragraph goes where. You won't have references at your fingertips or the opportunity for further research. That's all fine. There should be a coherent, critical discussion running through the writing, however.

Many exams will ask you to detail procedures and clinical decision-making (presenting a scenario and asking what you would do and in what order). You will obtain the highest marks for these questions if you do more than describe the necessary actions. Explain why you would do them, the underlying reasoning. It's also possible to discuss why you would prioritise in a certain way, what must be attended to first and what is less important initially. What if circumstances alter? Would that change your actions? The toddler and teenage questions are useful here too. Why (what are the reasons or evidence underpinning these actions)? So what (what might happen if you did not do this)? Suddenly, instead of writing a list you are composing an in-depth, critical discussion of the issues.

Taking a critical approach in presentations

By now, you will have noticed a theme emerging no matter the assessment: in the later stages of your degree, or to achieve the highest marks at any level, a critical approach is essential. This is equally true of presentations, a common assessment in any healthcare programme. It is far easier to tell stories than present a critical discussion within presentations, however, this is particularly true when you are nervous, or if you really don't like public speaking. So make sure you are not choosing the easy option. Be careful not to add too many flowery or irrelevant details to any talk you deliver. Consciously demonstrate your critical approach in presentations, as in anything else at university.

I think the two most important tips for presentations are:

1. Spend time planning and researching your presentation. This allows you to deliberately include critical elements within it and ensures you have a broad enough evidence base to talk through a topic in a knowledgeable manner. As with essays and longer exam questions, it also means you will stick to the task and construct a logical and convincing argument.
2. Practise your presentation. It is not usually a good idea to commit a presentation to memory – this is likely to come across as artificial and, if you forget any element of

it, you may become completely unstuck. You should definitely rehearse it several times, however. That way, you will have figured out your timings (at what point you should be on what slide). You should also feel more confident in the terminology and the sound of your voice discussing the topic.

People often forget that you require evidence and references in presentations, just as in other assessments. It is not always necessary to talk about them (and it would be a pretty boring presentation if you read out too many quotations and statistics followed by the author details). Instead, add them to your slides and handouts using the same referencing system as you would use for written work. Remember to also add reference details for any graphs, images or diagrams you take from published sources. This will add academic rigour to your discussion and allow you to cite convincing evidence for any claims you make.

Sometimes in presentations, you are asked to defend a particular position, argue for one side of a debate. This is to assess how well you can construct and present an argument. It is still possible to be critical, however. When undertaking your research, it can be worthwhile to initially take an objective approach to the topic and consider all perspectives. You will obviously want to present the evidence in favour of the side you have been given but it is great to know what your opposing presenters are likely to say. You also then have the opportunity to demonstrate your awareness of these competing perspectives and explain why they are less convincing than your own.

Mistakes in reasoning

Ad populum and received wisdom

Ninety-six out of 127 readers would recommend the shampoo to their friends.

Everyone knows that humans only use 10 per cent of their brain. Imagine what we could do if we harnessed all of it!

The first argument is an appeal to popularity – if so many people think something is good, then it must be true. Well that is not actually a logical argument. Lots of people can be wrong.

The second argument does something similar but argues from received wisdom. It does not present any evidence to support the case, relying instead on the fact that it is a popular belief (myth). There is lots of discussion about the 10 per cent myth but absolutely no evidence that it is true. In fact, brain imaging research suggests that we use most areas of the brain all of the time.

Notes on activity: recognising critical writing

Extract A

This extract is well written and uses a number of references to provide evidence for its main argument (a link between spirituality and health). It is more descriptive than critical, however. It doesn't do anything other than state the assertion.

Why might there be a connection between spirituality and health? Is there any way of explaining the results of the studies? Might there be any problems with the studies cited? Could there be alternative explanations or evidence that contradicts these findings?

It also doesn't draw any implications. What might this mean for healthcare? How could this knowledge be used in nursing practice?

Extract B

This extract provides a succinct description of the research – its aims, methods and findings. It then considers some problems with the paper and makes critical observations, using other references to substantiate points.

It also takes a critical approach in considering whether the findings are relevant in a UK context. It finds evidence to show that levels of religiosity and healthcare systems differ to such an extent that the results could well be very different if the study were replicated in Britain.

Extract C

This extract provides a rational argument for increased emphasis on spirituality within healthcare. It gives examples of what nurses could do, thus considering implications for practice. It also makes good use of policy and research. It could be improved by considering theory and trying to make sense of the evidence. Why might this link exist?

The main problem with this text is that it fails to consider alternative viewpoints or barriers to its recommendations. What might prevent a nurse from emphasising or prioritising spiritual needs? Time, training, concern about appearing ignorant or prejudiced? What about those patients who resent the intrusion? How would the impact of these changes be measured? Does this conflict with the current rationalist model of healthcare? What about economic constraints? In a time of limited budgets should money be spent on spiritual needs or are other concerns more of a priority (e.g. staffing, access to medicine)?

The piece would be much more critical and well-rounded if it presented multiple perspectives, the different sides of the debate. It could then, perhaps, side with one more than the others, so long as a justification for this was included.

Chapter 6

Taking a critical approach in literature reviews

Overview of chapter

Many assessments in the later years of a degree involve literature reviews, either as a stand-alone piece of work or as an introductory section of a dissertation or paper. This kind of assessment requires many of the skills you have been developing through the course of this book – critical engagement, questioning, selecting resources, for example. It is a unique type of assessment, however. It is all too easy to fall into the trap of taking a descriptive or superficial approach to the literature.

This chapter begins by defining literature reviews before detailing the distinct stages involved in the process of writing one. Finally, the chapter examines how to ensure a critical synthesis when writing literature reviews.

Learning outcomes

By the end of this chapter, you should be able to:

* recognise the purpose of a literature review;
* understand the separate stages involved and plan your activities when undertaking a review;
* evaluate literature reviews and construct your own from a critical perspective.

Writing critical literature reviews

What is a literature review?

The vast majority of degree programmes involve the writing of a literature review. For some, this will be the basis of an entire dissertation; for others, it will be the first chapter or the early part of a research paper. Either way, it is vital that you are able to demonstrate your critical thinking when writing it. If you don't, you haven't produced a literature review or systematic review but have simply provided a description of a number of different papers.

So, as with other assessments, it is really important to understand exactly what is being asked of you. If you read a really well written literature review, what should you have gained from it?

Table 6.1 Good vs bad literature reviews

A good literature review	A bad literature review
Tells you much more than if you simply read all of the papers yourself	Is little more than an annotated bibliography
Asks and answers an appropriate question – engages with a topic of sufficient breadth and depth	Is shallow, failing to really explore the topic and covering too narrow an issue
Is written in a logical and coherent manner	Appears to be written almost arbitrarily and is thus confusing to read
Uses rigorous and consistent research methods	Provides no information about methods or simply describes the literature search
Includes critical analysis – evaluating the strengths and weaknesses of the component papers	Does nothing more than describe the literature that has been located
Is a synthesis of the research – drawing out themes and making conclusions from the findings	

- a thorough understanding of the context of the topic (why it matters, the remit or scope, background and definitions)
- an outline of the methods used to find the literature and justification of the decisions taken during that process (search terms, exclusion criteria, …)
- an overview of the available evidence (published papers, relevant policy/procedures, grey literature)
- a critical synthesis of research on that topic (emerging themes, conclusions, evaluation of the methods and findings)
- a theoretical perspective (theories/models/frameworks that would assist understanding of this topic)
- an application of findings to your profession
- discussion of the limitations or gaps in the available research and suggestions as to the direction for future research.

A literature review should do so much more than summarise the contents of the papers it considers. It should, for example, critically evaluate those papers, synthesise the emerging findings and contextualise the information. It is much greater than the sum of its parts. That is a pretty big task, but you should be aiming to have the same impact. Does the reader gain all of that from your work? That is what the marker is looking for.

Unfortunately, it's all too easy to produce a lesser piece of work.

Activity: reading the literature review section of a paper

It is reasonably straightforward to become familiar with literature reviews. They are the beginning section of any research paper that you read. They are often indicated by a sub-heading of 'literature review' or 'background'. So take note of them. This will allow you to see how authors write about literature – the terminology, the structure, the different ways of engaging. Some reviews will discuss papers thematically, drawing out and separating the different aspects of the topic. Others may simply present what is known about the subject in a relatively chronological manner. The former method is likely to be more complex and fruitful. Some will critically engage with the literature they are discussing, noting similarities, strengths, outlying results or problematic elements. Others may summarise the findings or major themes. Whilst such a superficial approach may be because the literature review is very brief within the context of the overall paper, it may nevertheless impact upon your judgement of it.

1.   Choose three research papers that are currently relevant to your degree.
2.   Locate the section of each paper that contains the literature review.
3.   Read each review in turn, and in isolation from the rest of the paper.
4.   Assess the effectiveness of each review in critically examining literature in the field, providing a synthesis of current research and locating a gap that justifies the need for further research (and thus the remainder of the paper).
5.   Reflect upon what you can learn from these extracts for your own literature review. Remember you can gain as much from the weaker extracts as you can from those that are excellent examples of critical evaluation of literature. Sometimes, it is about recognising what to avoid. Very few pieces of published research are flawless.

The stages of a literature review

Literature reviews are like other assessments in the later stages of your degree. They require a great deal of autonomy or independence from you. Whilst support will still exist in the form of your tutors, lecturers etc., you are in charge of a lot more. You will make decisions as to the direction of your work, the eventual structure of the written piece and so on. Your topics of study will be much more specialised. This means that, whilst tutors can advise you, they may not be experts on the subject at hand. Increasingly, you will be the person who knows the issues best. The trick is to see all of these developments as empowering. You are becoming an independent practitioner. It is important to accept that this level of personal responsibility and decision-making is necessary when undertaking a literature review.

People can become quite stressed out by literature reviews because, at the beginning, they have no real idea what the finished piece of work will look like. With other assessments, it is possible to predict the overall structure. With an essay, for example, after some brief brainstorming and initial research, you can usually decide upon the three or four topics that will be discussed, as well as the natural order for that discussion. This is not normally the case for literature reviews. You won't know what the literature says about a topic until you have read it.

There are distinct stages to a literature review; and you cannot rush them or skip any. So, for example, you won't know the topics and structure until you have read the literature. But you can't read the literature until you have refined your topic of investigation. Everything must be done in a certain order. My advice is to recognise the distinct stages and accept that there will be periods where things seem quite unclear or amorphous. This is also part of the process: going in to uncertainty so that you can emerge, later, with your own distinct take on the issues.

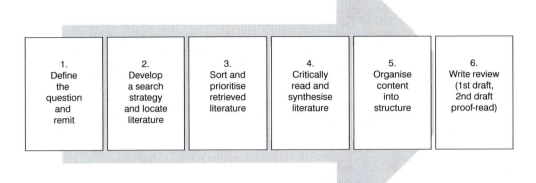

Figure 6.1 Stages of a literature review

Define the question and remit

You are likely to refine the details of your question and the precise remit or boundaries of your study as you progress. Perhaps you will find that there is a great deal of literature on some topics and very little on others, so you return to your question and refocus it. Or, perhaps, you discover that most of the work concerns a particular client group so you decide to narrow the range of the population you will consider. Nevertheless, it is important to spend time at the beginning working out exactly what you are attempting to investigate.

This first stage involves a fair amount of brainstorming and experimentation. So what research problem are you looking to answer? Is there a particular clinical issue you are seeking to examine? Have you been given a specific topic or question? It is often helpful to frame your research aim as a question. That way, you are likely to stay focused on actually answering it, rather than spending ages researching and writing about nothing in particular. It will also ensure you take a critical approach to the topic. As we've seen throughout this text, questions trigger greater critical engagement. Why is this the case? Why does this matter?

Next, you need to delineate the boundaries of your review. This is all about decision-making and being clear why you have made those decisions. What are the precise definitions you will be using? What is outside the boundaries of your research – things that are related and, perhaps, very interesting but you do not have the time or word capacity to include for this assessment? Think about parameters. Which questions are you going to be seeking answers for and which are outside of the confines of the review? Often, you can develop a much clearer understanding of what you are trying to do by explicitly acknowledging what you are not.

Develop a search strategy and locate the literature

Having worked out what you are aiming to find out, the next task is to develop a search strategy that will allow you to gather the research to answer your question. You will no doubt be considering these things whilst undertaking the first stage of the process, but they are separate tasks. So, first, decide upon your search terms. What words will you use to find literature on your chosen topics? Are there any synonyms you should be including? Are there international expressions you should be utilising? It is worth doing a little experimentation to check you are getting the kind of search results you would expect for those terms. This will let you know if you need to refine your terms or become more flexible. Be sure to make a note of all of your decisions and the reasons behind them. For critical engagement, it will be necessary to justify your choices and provide evidence to support them.

Next, decide which databases you will search. Again, be sure you are making rational choices you could justify to a reader. In the past, you may have relied upon your library catalogue and one or two journals in your field. For a literature review, you require current, empirical research so you will need to become comfortable searching electronic databases. There will be plenty of support available as you acquire this skill so take advantage of your librarians and learning support specialists. Many institutions have support staff who are able to take you step by step through your first couple of searches.

You will also need to devise inclusion and exclusion criteria as part of your search strategy. The development of your question and remit in the first stage will help you with this. Now you have some further criteria to determine, as you decide upon the volume and type of information you require. Ask yourself these questions, make a note of your decisions and remember to have critical reasoning underpinning your choices:

- Will you exclude certain kinds of interventions? If so, why?
- Will you exclude papers with certain kinds of research design? If so, why?
- Will you exclude certain categories of participants or populations? If so, why?

Box 6.1 Example notes of a search strategy

6th October – Lit review search strategy
Working title: The effectiveness of honey dressings in the treatment of pressure ulcers in the elderly

Search terms: honey, honey dressing, manuka honey, nursing care, nursing, wounds, wound care, pressure ulcers, gerontology, elderly care, anti-inflammatory, anti-microbial, bioactivity,

Use AND/OR/* Boolean terms

Medline

1. honey dressing – 101
2. honey dressing AND wound care – 56
3. honey dressing AND pressure ulcers – 9
4. pressure ulcers AND elderly – 140

- Which publication dates will you exclude? When do you consider research obsolete, too dated or superseded by later events? Why?
- Will you exclude papers from certain geographical areas? Are you only looking for UK-based work or might research from North America or Australasia be relevant? Why? Why not? What additional critical questions will you need to ask of international research and the socio-economic, political and cultural context from which it is derived?

It is likely that some of your inclusion and exclusion criteria will need to be tweaked once you begin searching for literature. Perhaps you have been too restrictive in your client group for example. If there is simply too little work involving young people, you may have to include those interventions involving adults and then draw out implications and parallels for a much younger client base.

Keep your overall literature review question, remit and search strategy near you as you search the literature. This will help you to stick to the task and will allow you to refine your search terms and inclusion criteria as you gain a more thorough knowledge of the subject area. It is at this point that you will get a sense of how reasonable your initial plans regarding the scope of the review were. Perhaps you will fail to locate enough relevant literature and should, therefore, broaden the scope. Or you may very quickly find that you are deluged by relevant material – there could simply be too many papers for you to manage within the confines of this particular assessment. If this is the case, it will be necessary for you to narrow your question and develop further exclusion criteria. This is a fortunate problem to have, however.

Activity: broadening or narrowing your literature review focus

A.   You have chosen an area of investigation and developed a search strategy, having decided to focus on *home-based falls prevention programmes for clients with Parkinson's disease.*

Unfortunately, no matter how many search engines or databases you use, you cannot locate sufficient literature on the topic. It seems there is simply not enough published research in this field. How might you broaden the scope of your review so that there is enough, credible literature? How might you exclude fewer papers?

B.   This time you are investigating *eating disorders in children*. You are overwhelmed by the number of papers that appear in your search results. How might you narrow the topic? Can you add exclusion criteria to refine your results?

There are notes on this activity at the end of the chapter.

At this point, you are well on your way to completing your literature review. You still won't have a full sense of the final shape of it, however. Your search strategy and the search itself will have shown you possible themes or subdivisions but you won't know these for sure until you have completed the reading, conducted your background research to understand the context of the main papers, and spent time planning. It is important to accept these limitations and not to try to force a structure on your review before you are ready. Your argument must emerge from your findings rather than trying to fit the evidence into your pre-planned conclusion or themes.

Sort and prioritise retrieved literature

You will obviously need to skim read papers as you locate them – look through the title, abstract, conclusion and references in full and glance over the other sections to determine relevance. Does this paper cover the material you expected it to? Does it meet any exclusion criteria that means it should be dismissed? If you decide it is worth reading in detail, it is often best to put it aside until you complete your literature search. If you read each paper immediately on locating it, you will not be separating the stages of the review. You are likely to become distracted and you may run out of time and have to begin writing up your assessment before you locate the truly relevant papers.

It can sometimes be difficult to stop searching, but you need to at some point. The anxiety is that, if you finish your search, you might miss out on important literature; the best paper could still be found if you keep plugging away. If you have been logical in your search criteria and have used all of the relevant databases and search engines, you can be confident that you have made every effort to find the available literature. There is, thus, no point in further searching. Again, it can be helpful to remember that literature reviews are completed in stages, but you need to move from one to another. If you find it difficult to leave this part of an assessment behind, perhaps try setting yourself a time deadline: by *date x* I will stop my literature search, prioritise papers and begin reading.

As you search, you are likely to begin sorting the papers into different categories/subjects/themes, mentally at least. Before you start reading in earnest, it's worth spending a little time completing that process. If you like print outs, physically sort them into different piles, if you prefer electronic versions, place them in different folders. This will allow you to prioritise your reading and to group subjects together. It makes sense to read everything about a particular topic at the same time, before moving on to the next one. You will build up a knowledge of the context and vocabulary the more you read about the topic.

Critically read and synthesise the literature

Think back to the chapter on reading literature. In particular, remember to:

- develop your critical reading questions and your literature review grid;
- keep some useful reference books or websites to hand;
- be prepared to do further research to understand the papers.

Reading the papers will be time consuming so set yourself a realistic deadline and keep at the task. Don't leave long periods where you are not engaged with reading for the review. Otherwise, you will quickly become unfamiliar with the subject matter. If you undertake the reading in regular chunks, you can develop an understanding of the methods, vocabulary and background to your topic.

Whilst you must necessarily read each paper as a stand-alone piece of research, and you need to evaluate it from that perspective initially, it is important to begin to consider the wider context whilst reading. Where does this paper fit within the broader knowledge base? How does it relate to the other papers you are reading? What does it have in common with them? How and why does it differ? And what does this mean for the subject and for practice? Make notes on these issues as well as the actual content of the paper – use literature grids or mindmaps to record these connections. This will ensure you are developing a critical synthesis of the literature.

Organise content into structure

Now, finally, you will be in a position to consider the thematic structure of the review. You can see why it is impossible to decide upon a plan or outline from the beginning. You simply don't know the content of the literature, and therefore the main findings and issues of discussion, until you have completed all of the earlier stages of the review.

Don't rush this aspect of the process, however. With any piece of critical writing, it is essential to spend adequate time planning: deciding upon the topics you will cover; the nature of that coverage and the logical order in which to introduce things. For longer assessments and for complex texts such as literature reviews it is particularly important. You will be examining difficult material and many different issues. If you have not worked out a meaningful way to present this information and critical discussion, your writing will appear chaotic. It may even seem like you do not understand the material about which you are writing.

The structure will be unique to your review, so you need to be confident and decisive. With essays, it is possible to ask for advice from colleagues who are also researching the issue, or tutors who are familiar with the subject area. Here, however, you are the expert on this literature and you need to make the decisions. Write as detailed a plan as you can and know at what point you will be covering each topic you wish to discuss.

There are likely to be several ways in which you can organise the material (by findings, by intervention type, chronologically). So long as you can justify your choice and there is an underlying logic behind it, your decision should be fine. Perhaps state explicitly why you chose to structure the review in the way that you did. That way, your reader will understand the decision.

Remember to begin by setting the scene, letting your reader know what is to come and why this is important. Provide context and any necessary background information and outline the structure of the rest of the work. It is also a good idea, at the planning stage, to consciously ensure you are taking a critical approach. Plan the review in a way that encourages you to synthesise the literature, to draw out the findings and discuss comparisons and relative strengths and weaknesses rather than taking each paper case by case.

Write the review

Some people like to write as they undertake their reading. Whilst it can be helpful to make detailed notes in your own words, I would recommend that you always delay writing the first draft of your assessment until you have completed your research. Otherwise, you won't have a full grasp of the topic and you won't have planned sufficiently. This is even more important with literature reviews, where it is necessary for you to undertake each of the elements of the process outlined above.

The good news is that, by completing your research and planning thoroughly, the writing part of the task should be more straightforward. Instead of a blank screen, you will have detailed planning notes and perhaps even literature review grids that bring all of the points together for you. You may still need to complete several drafts. This very much depends on whether you like to write quickly and then correct style and clarity later or whether you write in a slower, precise manner. Either way, you already know where the argument is going, where one section fits into the overall structure and what topic will be covered next. Most of the difficult decision-making has been undertaken. Your writing style should be the same as for other pieces of formal, academic writing. Aim for clarity and be sure to use signposts to allow your reader to follow your argument.

Activity: spot the deliberate mistakes

The extracts in Boxes 6.2–6.4 all display some kind of error that is occasionally made by students when writing literature reviews. Can you tell what the problem is? What is preventing it being a critical piece of writing? What could be done to correct the issue(s)?

There are notes on this activity at the end of the chapter.

Box 6.2 Example extract I

Introduction

This review examines literature concerned with modern nurse education, in particular papers that engaged with the challenges or issues faced by nurses immediately after registration with the Nursing and Midwifery Council and on taking up employment. Findings suggest that newly qualified practitioners lack confidence in both their clinical and theoretical knowledge and, whilst facilitated support such as mentors can be effective, further measures could be put in place to improve their experience and performance.

The review begins with an outline of the search strategy employed, before discussing the themes emerging from the literature.

Box 6.3 Example extract 2

Search strategy

In order to locate appropriate literature, a search was undertaken on relevant databases. These were EBESCO, CINAHL and Medline. For each, combinations of the terms 'nurse', 'education, 'training', 'development', 'university', 'preregistration' and 'undergraduate' were used to find papers. Titles and abstracts were read to determine relevance to the question. 56 papers were initially found and then narrowed down to 20. These were read and evaluated for inclusion in the review.

Theme I: widening access to the profession

Box 6.4 Example extract 3

Findings

Adams (2012) has argued that nurse education is still located in an awkward position between the traditional professions and domestic service. Whilst it is now taught within universities, it is not necessarily viewed as an academic discipline and faces hostility from both external critics, in the government and the media most notably, and from those within its own ranks.

Thomas (2009) undertook semi-structured interviews with 20 newly employed nurses within six months of their graduation. 90% indicated that they lacked confidence when acting alone and initially felt unprepared for full-time clinical practice ...

McDougall (2011) administered questionnaires to those supervising newly qualified staff nurses.

Top tips for literature reviews

1. Read other literature reviews. This might sound obvious, but do you know what a literature review looks like? You have probably read plenty of brief ones at the beginning of papers but have you scrutinised many of the longer versions? If not, it is well worth doing so. Literature reviews vary considerably because they are so dependent upon the particular topic and discipline. There is a general style and structure that you can discern, however. This will give you a feel for them and you will begin to have a clearer understanding of what yours might look like.

    It will be particularly useful to find some literature review models for your area of expertise. Hopefully, you won't find something on the exact topic that you are covering – there isn't much point in spending significant time on it, if it has already been done – but research moves on very quickly, so unless your topic was covered and published in the last six months, there is probably further work for you to discover.

2. Construct a working statement or question and amend it as you progress with the work. One of the things people can find difficult about literature reviews is the lack of guidance. Unlike an essay, you are not given a specific question to answer. And without a question, it can be easy to become side-tracked, to go off topic or simply wander from issue to issue with no real focus. That doesn't mean you can't write your own question, however.

    As soon as you begin framing your literature review questions and search strategy, draft a question or title to help you remain focused. This is likely to require refinement as you proceed. The parameters of your topic will change as you dig further into the literature and become aware of what has been explored and where the gaps remain, but simply amend your question when this happens. At the planning and writing stage, it will be particularly important to keep the question around you. This will help you develop your argument, stay on topic and actually have something meaningful to say. It is easy to get lost in the midst of writing, to forget what the point was in this sea of literature. Your question will act as a map. It will remind you what the purpose was, what you were trying to find out from the literature.

3. Read the easiest papers first. When you have completed your search and filtered the literature so that you are left with the ones that require close reading and evaluation, there are no rules about the order in which you must read them. It is up to you. So why not start with the ones you find easiest. This may be because you are familiar with the topic or research method, or perhaps because they are shorter or simply written. Whatever the reason, they are likely to lay a much better foundation to your understanding than some of the more complex papers. You will find the more difficult papers easier to get to grips with once you are experienced in reading about the topic.

4. Keep a diary of your progress. I don't mean a blog in which you pour out your heart and soul or express how difficult you are finding the task or how ground-breaking your findings are (though feel free to do that if it helps!). I mean a brief note of your decisions and reasons for them, as you undertake the literature review process. This will make life easier when it comes to writing up and it will ensure you have been logical and consistent in your literature searching. So keep a record of your search terms and word combinations, write down the databases you use, etc.

5. Decide upon a bibliographic filing system at the beginning of the process. Literature reviews, by their very nature, will require extensive reference lists and bibliographies. You will have your primary papers, the underpinning background references, the policy documents and so on. Where and how will you be recording all of their bibliographic details? You have a lot of options so it depends on your personal preference. There are plenty of electronic referencing systems – some can even upload all of the details directly from your database searches. With a few clicks of a mouse, and a proofread, you can automatically produce correctly formatted reference lists in the style required for your submission. Your institution will have information on which referencing software is available to you.

    Others prefer a more old school approach. When I was writing my PhD, I kept a card index box on my desk. This was alphabetised and there was a small card for each text I had read and thought I might require as a reference in the future. I noted the bibliographic details (authors, title, journal title, volume and issue number, page number …) and a couple of sentences detailing the contents. This proved invaluable as the number of texts grew. Whatever method you choose, make sure you begin making a note of the details in a systematic way early on.

6. Leave plenty of time for writing up. As discussed above, there are several stages to a literature review and these stages are rather self-imposed. You have to have the confidence and discipline to know when to stop one stage (e.g. decide that you have found all of the literature that you going to) and when to begin the next one. It is easy to blur the boundaries between them or fail to leave sufficient time for the latter ones. So, be strict. Planning and writing always take time, when done well. Make sure you have enough.

7. When proofreading, check that you do not have lots of paragraphs beginning with an author's name. This may be a bad sign. You are likely to be simply describing the research rather than analysing or synthesising it. Why are you covering each paper in turn? It is likely to be a much more critical piece of work if you discuss them side by side.

8. Don't forget the non-research literature or grey literature. Even though literature reviews are primarily an investigation of empirical research, you should use a variety of sources in your discussion. You cannot fully understand the impact of a piece of research or consider how its findings might influence practice unless you are aware of the legislative

context or perhaps even the cultural or financial one. This is where government policy or professional body publications and announcements should be considered.

Mistakes in reasoning

Causation versus correlation

Over the last 30 years, whenever the majority of European countries have a centre-right government in power, the average summer temperature has been lower than when centre-left governments are in charge. Therefore, one of the best ways to reverse climate change may well be to vote for more right-wing parties.

Research has consistently suggested that dog owners weigh less than those who do not own pets. Does owning a dog allow people to maintain a healthy weight more easily?

Just because two things happen simultaneously does not mean that one causes the other. It is very easy to conflate causation (one thing causing another) with correlation (two or more things occurring near to each other or at a similar point in time). In the first example, lower temperatures appear to have occurred at the same time as particular governments. This does not necessarily mean that those temperatures are caused by the political orientation of voters. It is hard to think of a logical reason why that would be so. In this case, it seems much more likely that there is a correlation between the two factors. In fact, it could be entirely coincidental and no longer true if recorded for another 20 years.

The second example suggests a connection between dog ownership and a healthy weight. Again, a direct causation seems difficult to prove and logically unlikely. Why would the act of ownership affect weight? How could metabolism change or diet be healthier purely due to ownership of a particular pet. Again, this appears to be a correlational relationship. Unlike the first example, however, there could well be a connection between the two events. Could other factors explain the relationship? Are dog owners more likely to take regular exercise in the form of dog walks, for example? And might this explain the lower weight? Often factors can have something in common, which is worth highlighting and exploring further. But make sure you are not attributing cause where none exists or where you cannot prove direct causation.

Notes on activity: broadening or narrowing your literature review focus

A home-based falls prevention programmes for clients with Parkinson's disease

It is possible to retain the elements of your original focus, the thing that interested you in the first place, whilst broadening it so that it can become viable as a literature review topic. At this point, you have narrowed your focus to such an extent, that you have effectively excluded the vast majority of research engagement that exists within this general area. So, widen it out somewhat. The overall topic is falls prevention programmes. You may find some research that evaluates home-based strategies but, perhaps, not enough. Consider other kinds of programmes in addition. You could then compare the effect of home-based ones against these alternatives. Another way to find results might be to search for programmes for broader groups, such as the elderly, or perhaps without specifying the client group.

B Eating disorders in children

This topic is far too broad. Of course there will be a huge number of papers that are related to the subject. Whilst you can still conduct a literature review on eating disorders, it is necessary to refine your focus. Might you concentrate on a specific disorder such as anorexia or bulimia? This is likely to reduce the number of search returns? Or it might be possible to limit the group. Could you investigate this issue in relation to adolescents or primary school children, perhaps young males? Are you interested in diagnosis, causes, treatment or prevention? This, again, will alter your search terms and refine your results.

If you find that you have too many papers retrieved from your literature search, the chances are you need to return to the earlier stages of the process. Go back and define your question and remit, reconsider your inclusion and exclusion criteria. This should help you refine your results and make things more coherent and manageable.

Notes on activity: spot the deliberate mistakes

The introduction

As this extract stands, it fails to provide any context for the review. Why did the author bother to search and evaluate the literature on this particular issue? Why should the reader care? Remember these reasons are not personal (that it is a topic close to your heart) but academic (that it has an impact on safe practice, that there are economic consequences, for example). It can be a really good idea to provide information about the nature of the review and to indicate your findings within the introduction, but don't forget to add background, provide definitions and parameters and explain why this all matters.

The search strategy

When conducting a literature review, it is necessary to make many decisions. Hopefully, these will have been based on sound reasoning. There will be a logic behind your choice of databases, the search terms employed, your exclusion criteria for dismissing certain papers. The problem with this extract is that it does not tell the reader about that reasoning. It describes what was done, but not why it was done. A well written, critical search strategy will explain the decisions and convince the reader that these were the most appropriate choices.

Findings

This extract fails to synthesise the papers that have been read. Instead, it appears to be detailing the contents of each paper, one by one, describing rather than critiquing. It is much better to write about the research within themes, discussing what they have in common and where they differ.

If you find that you are beginning each paragraph with an author's name or by starting to describe a new paper, the chances are you have fallen into this trap. Watch out for it when proofreading your work.

Chapter 7

Taking a critical approach in dissertations

Overview of chapter

Almost every degree programme involves the development of an extended piece of coursework, often called a dissertation. This is usually undertaken in the latter stages of your programme, when you have developed an in-depth knowledge of the field, advanced clinical skills and experience and a wealth of critical skills. These will all be necessary to write such a complex and independent assessment.

Through this book, you will have been practising and honing the latter group of skills and you will require them throughout the dissertation process. The design of the question, the review of literature, the research and the write up all require critical evaluation. This chapter considers the tasks involved in writing a dissertation and the importance of planning, using feedback effectively and making the most of your supervisor. It also provides hints on remaining critical and suggests a technique for staying focused and developing your academic writing.

Learning outcomes

By the end of this chapter, you should be able to:

- use planning techniques to break down tasks and set deadlines for the completion of your dissertation;
- understand the importance of the dissertation supervisor role;
- consider developing and updating a working abstract throughout the dissertation process.

The different kinds of dissertations

The dissertation is an extended piece of independent work. It is designed to test your self-direction and self-motivation as well as your research and writing skills. It also requires you to demonstrate an expert understanding of the subject matter at hand.

The precise form of your work will be dependent upon the programme and module. Sometimes, you are given several types of dissertation from which to choose. Some students conduct literature reviews, critical reviews or systematic reviews as their dissertation. These involve a review and critical evaluation of literature on a particular topic and is covered in detail in Chapter 6. For others, the final project will be an extended essay. Sometimes, students are asked to complete a research proposal. This might involve a literature review, a discussion of methods, participants, ethical issues, resources and a proposed timeline, everything but the research.

For many students, the dissertation involves the planning and completion of empirical research. You may develop a hypothesis, which you test by way of an experiment. This requires a review of the background literature, application to an ethics committee, the design and undertaking of research and finally analysis and discussion of the findings. Occasionally, it is possible for dissertation students to participate in existing research projects, working alongside researchers and academic staff as junior members of a research team.

Planning and your dissertation

It is likely that your dissertation is the biggest piece of coursework you have ever been required to produce. Whether the structure of your degree involves you undertaking the task in one semester or two, whatever the nature of your enquiry and the exact word limit expected, it is no doubt an enormous undertaking. This can seem rather daunting, even overwhelming, but don't forget that you are coming towards the end of your course. You have a wealth of knowledge and experience and there is likely to be plenty of support as you conduct your research and write up your dissertation.

One of the best ways of dealing with such a large task is to break it down into its smaller constituent parts. It is also important that you manage your time well and plan carefully. Often with a project as big as a dissertation, and a deadline as far away as it may appear when first considering it, people can react in one of two ways:

1. They consider how much work they have to do between then and now and become so overwhelmed that they cannot face the task. They avoid truly engaging with their dissertation, whilst regularly worrying about it.

OR

2. The deadline feels extremely far away which leads the student to think they have lots of time before they need to start work on the dissertation. They ignore it and, instead, concentrate on other aspects of their programme. Suddenly, months have passed by and there is actually very little time before the dissertation submission date.

Neither scenario is particularly conducive to the production of a strong, critical dissertation. Behaving in this way also tends to add stress and anxiety to your already very busy life. The solution is good planning, sticking to realistic deadlines and regularly engaging with the work.

Activity: the tasks involved

What are the different tasks involved in producing your dissertation?

*   Note down everything you have to do from being given the module handbook to your final submission.

- Now put them into chronological order. (What do you need to do first, second …? What is the final task?)
- Finally, think about timings. Can you set a deadline for each of those tasks? Try working on the deadlines by beginning at the end point. You know your submission date so you will want your final deadline to be a couple of days before that.
- You have now produced a detailed plan with deadlines for each subtask.

An example task plan

Task	Sub-tasks	Deadline
Arrange first supervision meeting		End of September
Devise research question	Brainstorm Scope literature	3 October

Whilst your task list might seem large, look at each individual element. None in isolation are that intimidating. You don't need to face the whole thing so long as you can deal with each little part. You've broken things down into manageable chunks and can set achievable deadlines to ensure you make progress at a regular rate.

There are notes on this activity at the end of the chapter.

Planning and time management

As we've seen, planning is tremendously important with such a big project. The above method is great for taking control of your dissertation, recognising the distinct elements and setting goals. There are other methods and useful tricks to allow you to stay on top of things.

One really helpful thing to do, at an early stage, is to map out the time you have in which to complete your dissertation. This will give you a visual sense of your deadline. It can be kept somewhere conspicuous to maintain your motivation and remind you of the task.

Whilst this is a good reminder and can provide you with the incentive to begin work if you have been procrastinating, the example in Figure 7.1 actually only features two elements of your life, however – the dissertation and Christmas. Few of us have such empty existences so it is necessary to plan your dissertation alongside your other activities.

Consider the other modules and assessments you have to complete over the same time period. Again, it is useful to plot these out somehow. Try using a planner to note the various deadlines you have (assessments, class tests, etc.). As a student, it is often easiest to plan according to semesters/trimesters rather than using an annual planner.

October			November				December					January				February				March					April	
14	21	28	4	11	18	25	2	9	16	23	30	6	13	20	27	3	10	17	24	3	10	17	24	31	7	14

Today   Formative   Christmas   Final
                                    hand-in   hand-in

Figure 7.1 Visually representing your dissertation deadline

	Jan5	Jan12	Jan19	Jan26	Feb2	Feb9	Feb16	Feb23	Mar2	Mar9	Mar16	Mar23	Mar30	Apr6
Mon			PIP class test											PIP group presentation
Tues								My birthday						
Wed											MCD4 reflective essay			Job application deadline
Thurs														
Fri					MCD4 essay due	Hen night				1st chapter feedback returned		Portfolio due		Dissertation!!!!
Sat		Work		Work	Work	Work	Work	Jill's wedding		Work	Work	Work		
Sun	Work		Work		Work	Work	Work		Work		Work		Work	

Figure 7.2 An example semester planner

Time	Monday	Tuesday	Wednesday	Thursday	Friday	Saturday	Sunday
8.00–9.00							
9.00–10.00							
10.00–11.00							
11.00–12.00							
12.00–13.00							
13.00–14.00							
14.00–15.00							
15.00–16.00							
16.00–17.00							
17.00–18.00							
18.00–19.00							
19.00–20.00							
20.00–21.00							

Figure 7.3 A weeky planner

In the example Figure 7.2, the student has noted all of their degree commitments in the coming months (essay deadlines, class tests, presentations and the dissertation deadline). This allows them to plan their time across the whole programme. There is no point in completing your dissertation on time and to a high standard if you are late with the other two essays or have failed to adequately prepare for an assessed presentation.

Remember, you don't undertake your studies in isolation. The rest of your life continues and you need to manage all of it – taking care of your children, keeping up friendships, earning money, even enjoying yourself every now and then. So is there anything outside of university that you should note in a planner? The above example shows work shifts that rule out study on those particular days. It also highlights an upcoming wedding that will require time and commitment. Fitting all of this in is perfectly possible, but it takes a little bit of planning. If you know you will be away for a few days, put it in to your schedule. Give yourself a deadline for immediately beforehand and increase your work rate in that week. That way, you will feel that you have earned the break and can enjoy it without feeling guilty.

Once you have an idea of how the semester looks, what you need to do and when, you can set deadlines for the smaller elements of the tasks. Then, each week, try planning your activities in detail.

Figure 7.3 shows an example weekly planner.

Feedback

One of the main things that makes a dissertation different from other forms of assessment, is that it is a 'work in progress' for quite some time. It is a piece of writing that you redraft, change and improve before finally submitting. With other work, you may not spend that much time redrafting. In fact, usually, you complete the task, submit it, receive feedback and then move on to the next assessment. With the dissertation, you are likely to have several opportunities to receive detailed feedback prior to submission of your final draft. It is really important to take advantage of this, but using feedback effectively takes a bit of work.

Consider when you have received feedback in the past. The most obvious place this has occurred is in *written feedback on essays and assessments*. In my experience, people are almost entirely concerned with whether they have passed or failed, and what mark they received. They rarely spend much time reading or considering the written feedback. Whilst that is understandable, it is important to also attend to these written comments. They will explain why you received the mark you did and it is this information that will allow you to learn from the assessment and improve your future work. There are other, less obvious, forms of feedback and they all provide opportunities to learn and develop your critical abilities:

- *Verbal feedback* during tutorials and conversations with academic members of staff. Feedback does not have to be written. When you discuss issues during tutorials or answer questions, you will be told whether you are on the right lines or if your argument is well constructed and sufficiently evidenced.
- During discussions *with peers*. Feedback is not only given by staff. Your fellow students may often tell you, perhaps indirectly, if they agree with you, if your argument is sound and if they are aware of other issues that are relevant to the topic.
- *At work* including performance reviews, interviews, applications. People regularly provide you with information about your performance. Feedback is not only given in an academic context.

Activity: feedback and you

We have established that you receive feedback in lots of different ways. It is worth reflecting on how you tend to deal with it. Think about one particular time in which you received feedback and answer the following questions:

1. What kind of feedback was it?
2. Who gave it to you?
3. How did you react? How did you feel?
4. Did it help you to learn? Did you understand it? Could you see what the person meant? Could you relate it to your assessment (if it was academic feedback)?
5. Did you act on it? Did you do anything as a result?
6. And finally, the most important question, does that tell you anything about how you have used (or failed to use) feedback in the past?

You will receive lots of feedback during your dissertation, from your supervisor, peers, any subject experts you contact. It is important that you react to it in a constructive manner. Understanding the purpose of feedback, the many and varied forms in which it is given, and the ways in which you have tended to react to it in the past, will help you get the most from it.

Tips for getting the most from your feedback

- Do not react emotionally. The comments are about the work, not you (nor your capabilities, understanding or the effort you put in to it). Negative remarks are not a reflection on you. It is simply advice on how to change/improve your dissertation.

- Look back over the work referred to in your feedback. Can you see what they mean? You might not be used to doing this. In the past, by the time you received feedback, you had finished the piece of work. So it might not have seemed worthwhile going back through your essay to understand the points that were being made. Now it is essential you do it (and, in fact, it is a really useful practice for any assessment).
- The chances are, when you submit a dissertation chapter, you are reasonably confident it is a decent piece of writing (why hand it over to be scrutinised otherwise). So, if you are told that further work is necessary, or that parts of it require change, it is natural to feel disappointed. Give yourself some time to recover, but don't wallow. Before too long, begin going through the revisions.
- If anything is unclear about the feedback (you don't understand the terminology, or you disagree, for example) ask for clarification.
- If it seems like the person giving you the feedback has missed the point, there is a problem with the writing not the marker. Strong, critical writing makes the argument absolutely explicit to the reader, leaving no room for misinterpretation or misunderstanding. If someone has failed to understand what you are trying to say, you have not stated it clearly enough. This in itself is feedback. Use it by returning to your work and making your writing more clear.

I have marked lots of essays and given plenty of feedback. I am an editor of a national journal so I read many papers and reviews and have to provide feedback to authors. Alongside that, I have written journal papers, chapters and books and, thus, have received quite a bit of feedback too. In my experience, 99 times out of 100, feedback and the ensuing revisions made to a piece of work, improve it. Everyone finds it difficult to hear less than glowing comments but it gets much easier when you see it as a constructive element of the dissertation process. Your final draft will end up substantially better than your earlier drafts as a result.

Making the most of your supervisor

Providing feedback is just one of the roles your dissertation supervisor will perform. The way you will be assigned your supervisor, the number of times you will be able to see them and how much of your work they will read and provide feedback on will vary according to your degree and university. This should all be made clear to you within module handbooks, etc. If it isn't, ask for the information. It is important that you understand the nature of the relationship and the expectations on both you (as a student) and on your supervisor (as someone there to provide support for your dissertation).

Supervisors cannot write the dissertation for you, and they are not there to make the content and structure decisions. They are an extremely useful resource, however. So what do supervisors offer?

It is in your interest to make the relationship work. You do not need to begin a lifelong friendship. You don't even have to particularly like the person, but it is important that you have a productive professional relationship. An effective supervisor can improve your dissertation immeasurably, making the process, your experience and the final product far better. Hopefully it won't be too difficult for you. Dissertation supervision tends to be one of the most rewarding parts of a lecturer's job so it is something people are quite happy to do.

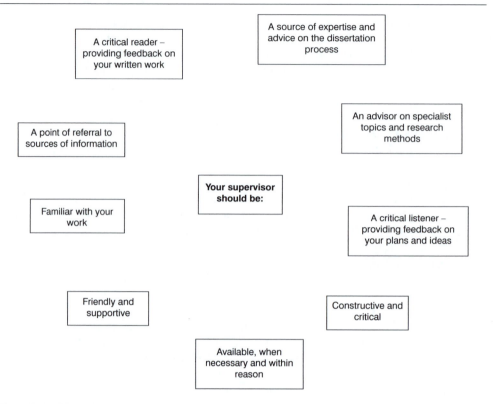

Figure 7.4 Your supervisor

There are a few things you can do to ensure a smooth relationship:

1. Be honest and communicative. Keep your supervisor up to date with progress. It can be tempting to avoid them if you are coming up against barriers or, perhaps, you have not been putting in as much effort as you meant to. But they are likely to be a source of advice when things are difficult. Admit you have fallen behind or that you can't locate sufficient literature and they might well be able to provide a solution for you.
2. Arrange your meetings in advance. They can be a useful deadline to impose upon yourself. So, for example, set up the meeting and let your supervisor know you will be bringing along your introduction. We are often better at making ourselves do something if we have told someone else to expect it.
3. Leave plenty of time for your supervisor to read your work. They will be extremely busy and cannot put everything else aside (their teaching, research, other marking, conferences, home life) simply because you have emailed them with a chapter. You have every right to expect a certain level of engagement from your supervisor but be reasonable in those expectations. If you need to have something returned to you by a specific date, make sure you submit it to your supervisor at least a few weeks in advance. It also makes sense to agree on a likely return date together.
4. When you contact your supervisor or attend a meeting with them, make sure you have specific questions or areas you wish to discuss. They cannot really help if you

arrive at their door saying 'aaarrrrgggghhhh, I'm stuck!' about every aspect of the dissertation. If you go along with a particular problem regarding a research paper or a dilemma as to which of two structures you should use, your supervisor will be able to understand your difficulty and offer advice.

Generating your question

Sometimes, the hardest part of a dissertation is the initial decision making. As with literature reviews, you are not usually given your research question. It is for you to devise and make of appropriate depth and critical possibility (i.e. it must be worthy of research and contain issues that can be subject to critical discussion, but not so broad that you remain on the surface and try to cover too many topics).

If you are at that stage in your dissertation, use the following questions to help think about your proposed work. Even if you are further along in the process, it is still worthwhile going through them. The questions offer a method of reflection, a way to pause and revisit your intentions and progress.

- What is the general topic you are investigating?
- Is there a specific focus?
- Why does this particular subject matter? Why bother researching it?
- Are you intending to write a literature review, research proposal or conduct a piece of research?
- Will you be examining a specific treatment or intervention?
- Are you investigating a particular client group?
- Is there a specific location e.g. acute setting, community?
- What kind of research are you hoping to find or conduct (quantitative, qualitative)?
- What do you think your findings are likely to be?
- What does this mean for professional practice?
- Which theories are likely to be relevant?
- Does this have implications for multi-disciplinary working or other professions?
- Can you draw on research or theories from other disciplines (sociology, psychology, medicine)?
- What policies and legislation are involved in this topic?

Spend some time brainstorming these questions. It can be helpful to talk them through with colleagues and, of course, your supervisor. Conduct some scoping research to gauge the amount and quality of research, policy and theory that is available in your chosen field. Above all, make decisions.

All of the planning work discussed above demonstrated that there is finite time in which to complete this assessment. It is imperative that you define the task quickly so that you can get on with the bulk of the research and the write up. In my experience, people can get somewhat stuck at the very beginning of the dissertation process. They become paralysed with indecision, unable to settle on one topic. It is easier to keep two or three topics as possibilities rather than making a final decision on the one you will definitely be researching. Take your time making the right decision, by all means, but give yourself a deadline. At some point, you will need to get on with it.

Tips to ensure a critical approach in dissertations

There is no secret formula to ensure your dissertation is critical. Instead, harness all of the skills you have developed through the course of your degree and clinical placements. Utilise all of the critical abilities that have been discussed in the book, from a general critical attitude, to reading and writing critically, to developing a credible argument (thesis) with convincing evidence (premises). Your dissertation will be a long piece of work and requires an explicitly critical approach throughout. It is never very effective to artificially introduce a critical argument towards the end of a piece of writing. This is even truer of dissertations. Your critical abilities must shine through in every section.

- Remember to explain and justify all of your decisions. Why this question? Why this research design? Why this analysis? Why did you dismiss other ones? Substantiate your decisions with evidence or logical reasoning.
- Remember to respond to feedback positively. The first draft you hand to your supervisor is just that, a draft. They may ask you to change a fair bit of it but don't be disheartened.
- Think about your writing style and structure. With longer assessments, it can be easy to lose your reader. They can forget where they are in your argument, what the overall topic or current subtopic is. So signpost things and add in summaries at appropriate points.
- Avoid lengthy descriptions and surface writing. This is tempting with larger assessments – you have a greater word count and can become anxious about filling it, with anything at all. You are not demonstrating your understanding or critical thinking by regurgitating huge chunks of description though. Instead, be discursive. You will find you have much more to write when you critically discuss the topic as there will be several perspectives to cover as well as their underpinning evidence, or lack of it.
- Consider diagramming your overall argument and sub-arguments. Once you have completed all of your research and are planning your write up, be sure you are clear on your main point. What is the overall purpose and findings, and why? Then think of the smaller arguments that build in to the bigger picture.

Writing a working abstract

As your dissertation is such a big undertaking, it can be easy to lose your way. You can go off topic, feel like you are not making any progress or that you don't know anything more about the subject than when you began your project. This is both time consuming and demotivating. There is a particularly effective trick for avoiding some of these issues, however. It may sound a little strange at first, but I have found that it really helps students produce critical pieces of work. In the early stages of your dissertation, whilst brainstorming or during the initial literature search, write an abstract.

An abstract is the paragraph or two at the beginning of any research paper. It provides an overview of the contents and is an effective way of quickly telling if a paper is worth further reading. Most dissertations also require an abstract. The exact requirements, in terms of word count, content, etc., may well be specified for you so check your module handbook or dissertation details. Most are several hundred words and are placed at the front of the submission, immediately after the title pages.

Abstracts are a short, clear summary of the project. A well written abstract will have given sufficient information to explain the research and findings as well as the reasons why this is important. It should leave the reader wanting to engage with the rest of the paper/dissertation, but it should be possible to read the abstract independently, so that it makes sense in isolation from the bulk of the writing.

Many people leave their abstract until last, as the final piece of writing in any project. This need not be the case, however. It can be fruitful to construct a working abstract, one you write very early on in the process. This will not be the final abstract you submit, as there is likely to be substantial redrafting required as you undertake your research. Instead, it is a handy, brief reminder of the aims and expected outcomes of your project. This has three distinct advantages that make the effort worthwhile:

1. It helps you remain focused. Whenever you feel like you have lost your way or you cannot articulate what it is you are attempting to do, you can turn to your abstract to remind yourself. With essays, it is a good idea to keep returning to the essay question and guidance to keep you on track and producing the work you have been asked for. This is not possible with dissertations since you are setting the question. So, you can use your working abstract in much the same way.

2. It helps to develop your writing. Abstracts require a precise writing style, one that prioritises formality and clarity. It is necessary to convey a great deal of complex information in a very short space. Practising writing in this way, hones your style. It makes you concentrate and decide on the vital information as opposed to the extraneous details. These skills will translate into the rest of your writing, improving all of it.

3. It helps you keep track of your learning. If you return to your working abstract at regular intervals, you will be reminded of your intentions and can see how your work has developed and progressed. You can redraft your expected outcomes or add in detail now that your findings are clearer. This is important from a motivational point of view. It is often difficult to see or feel progress when you are in the midst of a challenging task, so this will demonstrate it for you.

Your series of working abstracts will also function as a record of your thinking or theorising through the project. Perhaps your eventual findings and recommendations are significantly different to those you had originally anticipated. This, in itself, can be useful to note, both from a personal, reflective point of view and for critical discussion in your write up. What lay behind your initial expectations? Why did it turn out differently?

In addition, the development of a working abstract is useful as a way of explaining your project to others in a succinct, well-rounded way. You can share the abstract with your supervisor, colleagues and others from whom you may be seeking advice or information. And, finally, it is a worthwhile exercise because, ultimately, you will be required to produce the abstract as part of your written submission. Whilst your working abstract is just that, a working statement, it will be possible to use it as the basis for your final version. You will have made a significant start on your final abstract.

Activity: composing your working abstract

Write a working abstract for your dissertation, or any other assessment on which you are currently working. Use the guidelines you have been given where appropriate. If you do not have any specific guidance regarding the abstract, make it 300 words in length.

It must contain:

- an outline of the aims;
- why the project is important;
- how you went about it (or plan to go about it);
- what you found (or what you expect to find);
- recommendations (or your anticipated recommendations).

You must use clear and precise language and ensure that your conclusions and recommendations fit the evidence.

If you find it difficult to write, go through research papers you have been using recently and critically read their abstracts in isolation. Note the language and content. Ask yourself if they fulfil the brief.

There are notes on this activity at the end of the chapter.

Return to your working abstract and update it regularly through the dissertation process.

Mistakes in reasoning

Representing all sides of an argument equally

Whilst Fosser and Barret (2015) and Schwarz (2014) argue that the link between excessive eating and obesity is clear, Patrick (2011) has claimed that a high body mass index is related to the type of housing the person occupies.

Several treatment options exist: the regular application of honey dressing (Taylor, 2009), a course of antibiotics (Martin, 2014), cleaning with sterile water (Jane, 2011) and one researcher (Trevor, 2012) argues for the use of crushed snails.

It is obviously important to discuss the different angles of an issue, the contrasting opinions or perspectives, but you must do this in a balanced way. You should not give every side equal weight because they may not all deserve it. In the above examples, the writer seems to be implicitly suggesting that both sides of the argument have equal merit or that the different treatment options are equally valid.

Is this really the case? Surely there is a great deal more evidence linking obesity to diet than to style of house. That should be reflected in your description. You may have good reasons for mentioning the other theory but it is important you add a note of evaluation or you make clear that very few others support such a stance. In the second example, the suggestion to use snails may have been published but is it worthy of mention? There will always be a variety of opinions and some will be controversial, experimental or downright wacky. It is worth considering whether you need to include them all. If they have no supporting evidence whatsoever, it may be appropriate to leave them out of your writing.

The press often like to include all sides to a debate, sometimes in pursuit of a fair hearing for all, sometimes so they can include controversial or extreme views to garner attention.

Notice when this is happening and evaluate whether the report is being representative of the relative weight of the views or theories under discussion.

Notes on activity: the tasks involved

If your dissertation involves empirical research, your task list might look like this:

- Decide on topic
- Define search terms and inclusion/exclusion criteria
- Conduct literature search
- Design research question and research instruments
- Complete ethics form
- Decide on methodology
- Conduct pilot and recruit participants
- Undertake data collection
- Transcribe results
- Analyse findings
- Write outline plan of structure
- Write detailed plan for each chapter
- Write introduction
- Receive and understand formative feedback
- Draft chapters
- Redraft/edit
- Complete reference list and bibliography
- Proofread
- Check against marking criteria
- Layout/presentation issues

As you note the tasks, they are unlikely to all occur to you in the exact order in which they need to be completed. The list above requires a bit more work to ensure everything is undertaken in the correct order. After that, it is simply a case of setting yourself deadlines (some of which may run concurrently – so you could be completing your literature review and developing your research instruments at the same time).

Notes on activity: composing your working abstract

Even though you may be very unsure about how your project is going to develop, the drafting of a working abstract is an enormously useful exercise. At the outset of your research, you should be clear about your aims and objectives, the academic motivations behind the project and the intended methods. If you cannot articulate these within an abstract, you need to spend a little time making things clearer to yourself, perhaps in discussion with your supervisor.

You may need to include some guesswork and speculation if you are at an early stage. So don't worry if you find that you are writing 'it may be', 'it could be', 'if results mirror others'. Return to the abstract later when you have concrete details and amend the wording.

Chapter 8

Taking a critical approach in reflection and reflective assessments

Overview of chapter

Reflection and reflective writing are both important aspects of modern healthcare practice. You will be expected to undertake reflective activities at every stage of your education and career. Many of the subsequent written pieces of reflection will be assessed as part of your coursework. As with other assessments, a critical approach is necessary to lift your thinking and writing above mere description or regurgitation. In reflective work, you have to be critical in your attitude towards the subject matter, reading and theory but it is also essential that you are able to fully critique your own actions, feelings and attitudes. This chapter will examine the basics of reflection and reflective writing and discuss ways of ensuring you achieve a critical perspective.

Learning outcomes

By the end of this chapter, you should be able to:

- recognise the features of reflective writing;
- use questioning to encourage you to reflect at a deep level;
- understand the difference between critical reflection and descriptive or surface reflection.

The basics – what is reflection and why do I need to do it?

You are, more than likely, familiar with the process of reflection. It is a major feature of most healthcare programmes and a significant aspect of professional practice. It is worth reminding yourself of the purpose and core principles, however.

At its simplest, reflection is thinking about a situation and your place within it in a conscious, structured manner. The aim in doing so is to:

- consider the evidence base behind what you are doing in order to better understand it;
- think about and analyse your actions, and the reasons behind them, in order to improve your professional practice;
- explore and explain events rather than simply describe them;

The incident (an event that you wish to explore)

Reflection will allow you to develop your understanding in several, interlinked ways

Step 1: explore the incident	Step 2: explore your feelings/behaviour/ reactions/assumptions	Step 3: relate the issues to relevant theory and evidence
This allows you to thoroughly determine the sequence of events, the actors involved, the physical context and any environmental factors that might have had an impact	This helps you understand your actions and learn from them for the future	This helps you understand why things happened as they did

Figure 8.1 Linking theory and practice

- analyse your anxieties, errors and weaknesses as well as your strengths and successes;
- determine what action you should take or knowledge you should acquire to improve your performance in the future.

Anything that can achieve such understanding and growth must be a deep and complex activity.

Unfortunately, it is easy to remain superficial or fail to critically reflect. We all mull over events. We think about our performance and may even evaluate how we acted in a particular circumstance. That is not true reflection, however. Don't be fooled into thinking that it is an easy activity or that you can get away with simply narrating what happened and throwing in a few feelings along the way. Proper reflection takes conscious effort and structure, a critical approach and maybe even some discomfort as you really try to understand your motives, actions and attitudes, and those of others around you.

One of the greatest benefits of critical reflection is that it allows you to link theory and practice. This is challenging – connecting your academic learning from texts and lectures to your clinical and placement experience – though it is essential that you integrate the two if you are to become a professional healthcare practitioner.

Having undertaken critical reflection and linked theory to practice you will have developed a much broader perspective. You will have examined the experience from different viewpoints, rather than simply your own. You will have demonstrated an awareness of the evidence and knowledge base from which you were working (or on which you need to develop your understanding). You will have searched for meaning in the events rather than simply trying to come to terms with them. Finally, you will have perceived your experiences within a much broader context.

As you've probably noticed, this is exactly what has been asked of you in critical thinking. It is the kind of engagement and activity that we have been discussing in earlier chapters. But it is important to be aware just how easy it is to complete a reflective exercise without critically reflecting. It is perfectly possible to undertake Step 1 in Figure 8.1, or even Steps 1 and 2 and believe that you have completed the task. You need to ask difficult questions and understand the issue from a broad, theoretical perspective to truly engage (Step 3).

Activity: the toddler and teenage questions in reflection

Chapter 2 introduced the idea of toddler and teenage questions to ensure you take a critical, questioning approach in everything you do. This works just as well for reflection.

- Think of a critical incident and very quickly describe it (either aloud or in note form). *I was given some feedback on my performance and was told that my role was likely to change in the future. I became tense and couldn't hide my feelings. It was obvious to my mentor that I was really upset and this completely mortified me.*
- Now keep asking yourself the toddler question – why? This allows you to begin to probe much deeper into the situation, your actions/reactions/assumptions/behaviours. If you ask why about the other people involved, it may also provide insight into their perspective. *Why did I react in that way? Why did I get so upset about a change in role? Why couldn't I hide my feelings? Why was I embarrassed that someone knew how I felt? Why couldn't I have talked it though instead of trying to hide it?*
- Finally, ask the teenage question – so what? This puts the situation into a wider context. You can begin to explore theory, search for meaning in the event and perhaps draw upon research or other knowledge to better inform your understanding. It can also be quite useful to gain a bit of perspective. It is easy to overestimate your role within an event or be too harsh on yourself (you are the centre of your universe but not the centre of *the* universe, 'so what?' makes sure you remember that). *So what that my mentor noticed that I was upset? So what that I find feedback on performance and professional change stressful? So what that my performance was not as incredible as I had hoped it would be?*
- This kind of questioning should lead to further questions that encourage you to engage with literature. *Is this a common issue amongst newly qualified professionals? What kind of support or personal development would alleviate this?*

Using models of reflection

If you are already part way through your healthcare degree, you are probably very familiar with using models to support your reflection. If not, there are plenty of useful resources available to improve your knowledge and understanding in this area.

There are many reflective models around to help guide you through the reflective process. They ensure you do not become stuck at a particular point on that journey. This is important because it is easy to only partially complete the process. There are a couple of stages where this is more likely to happen:

- Some people become stuck on the story. They tell it in such detail there is no space for anything else.
- Others go wrong when it comes to the incorporation of feelings. They make the reflection only about them (self-justification, rants and self-pity or, perhaps, far too harsh a judgement or unrealistic expectations). Whilst it is vital that you consider

your feelings, reflection should remain a professional activity rather than a diary entry. It also needs to look beyond your own perspective, to the wider, theoretical implications and evidence, and to the views and actions of others in the situation.

• Some fall at the final hurdle. Having evaluated and searched for meaning, they forget to consider their learning for the future or to create a realistic action plan.

Reflective models are organised so that you do not trip up at these points. They ask questions that guide you through or they are structured to specifically include consideration of learning plans, for example.

Whilst models are useful in getting you to undertake critical reflection, how they do that differs. Some are very detailed, with lots of questions and sections. This can be great if you wish to be led through the exercise but some people may find such an approach restrictive. Other models seem to have fewer elements and thus grant a little more freedom to the individual. It is important to remember that they require just as much from you, however. Some models put great emphasis on your feelings, others less so.

When you are given a choice about which model to use, think carefully about it. Don't simply stick to the ones you always employ, conduct some research and experiment with other models. You may find one that is much more suited to your learning preferences, or even the particular reflective assessment you have been given.

Reflective writing

So what are markers looking for when they give you a piece of reflective writing to submit?

1. Most importantly, they are expecting you to have undertaken sufficient depth of analysis – far more than simple description. Rather than simply detailing how you felt and behaved, you should aim to explain *why* you felt and behaved in that way. Or consider the experience from all viewpoints – investigate each actor and what might explain their perspective.

2. They wish to see honesty – considered, critical evaluation of your actions, feelings, assumptions, behaviour, etc. What did the incident tell you about yourself? What was surprising? What might explain those feelings and beliefs? Were you correct in your thinking and assumptions? In hindsight had you over-reacted?

3. Ideally, you will consciously demonstrate the learning you have gained both from the incident and the reflection that was subsequently undertaken. What do you know now that you didn't before; how have you developed as a practitioner; what would you do differently?

4. Finally, it is important to consider and write about your plans for the future. In some models, and in some assessments, you will be expected to provide a detailed action plan involving SMART targets (specific, measurable, achievable, relevant and time-bound). In any case, be realistic about what you need to do, how you will go about it and how you will recognise when you have achieved it.

Characteristics of reflective writing

Whilst there are some important differences between reflective and academic writing, the two styles have much in common. Practising one is helpful in developing your style with the other. For both, the most important issue is to get your point across in a clear, precise, formal manner. Aim for maximum clarity rather than over-the-top vocabulary.

The main differences to academic writing are:

- You might use the first person rather than the passive voice that is expected in standard academic writing (I felt that, I began my shift, my confidence levels were high).
- You will be writing about your personal experiences. This is completely inappropriate in academic writing when you would not refer to your own circumstances or events in your life.

These changes may feel awkward but they become easier with practice and some people find that they really enjoy the personal element involved in reflective writing. You are still writing a formal piece of assessed work, however. And so, a balanced vocabulary is necessary. Lengthy descriptions should be avoided and make sure you do not become informal or chatty in style (this is very easy to do when discussing issues concerning yourself – it's how we talk to one another).

Structure in reflective writing

As with other written assessments, it is essential that you consider the structure of any reflective writing you submit. There should be an introduction, main body and summarising conclusion. It is best to decide all of this in advance and write a detailed plan. Reflective models can often provide an obvious structure, especially for shorter pieces of writing. In the main, writing based on models will have three separate sections:

The what	A description of what happened in as succinct a way as you can. Include pertinent details (everything the reader needs to know to understand the rest of the work) but rein in this section as much as possible. It is so easy to provide unnecessary details or concentrate on shallow description. So, cut out as much as you can. The vast majority of your word count should be used for the two boxes below.
The why	What might explain things? Search for meaning in events, evaluate your actions and feelings, relate to theory and look for evidence to better understand the context.
The what are you going to do about it	This section will outline your plans for the future. What do you need to do or learn, how are you going to do it, when and what measure of success will you use (how will you know when you have achieved what you set out to do)? What can you realistically accomplish and why do you think this is the case? How will this help?

For longer assessments, it may not be appropriate to use a simple structure that follows the exact pattern of a reflective model. If, for example, you have been asked to reflect upon your development of a particular skill over a period of years, perhaps with reference to items within your professional portfolio, it will not make any sense to use the structure above. Work out the most appropriate way to tell the reflective story you are trying to convey. You may wish to describe, evaluate and explore each aspect of that development in turn. Perhaps you begin with a critical incident involving your first interaction with that skill before moving to events in later years of your programme. You, thus, have a series of incidents that you wish to reflect upon individually before moving on to an analysis and evaluation of your performance, knowledge, behaviour and feelings over time.

For something as complex as this, it would be difficult and unhelpful to follow the exact structure of a model too precisely. It would not fit with what you were trying to explain. Think carefully about the structure of your reflective writing and write a plan before you start your first draft.

Activity: evaluating reflective writing

Read the extracts below and evaluate their effectiveness as pieces of reflective writing. What are their strengths? Could they be improved? Are there any limitations?

The presentation

By the time it came to my section of the presentation we had nearly used up all of our allocated time. I think this probably added to my nervousness and led to me speaking even quicker than I usually do. I kept tripping over my words and losing my place. Even though the slides had most of the details on, there were a few vital points I forgot to mention.

I felt really disappointed in my performance. I had spent a long time researching the topic and was confident that I could demonstrate sound understanding, but this did not come across in my presentation. I plan to work on my presentation skills to improve my public speaking in the future. I will be less nervous and try not to rush through talks as much.

The group task

We were given a group task by the tutor for our inter-professional learning module. This was the third module of the year and the one I liked the least if I am honest. Each member of the group was to choose an area of the problem to research and we all had to put the information together on a wiki. We were going to be given individual marks for our contribution and an overall team mark, which would be divided by the number of people within the group. In addition, we would mark each other and this would count for 10 per cent of our result.

As a team we started off well but things soon became tricky. When we met after lectures in the café nearby not everyone turned up on time and two people in the group kept making excuses for not doing the work they were supposed to have.

There are notes on the extracts at the end of this chapter.

Critical reflective writing

True reflection *is* critical. If you haven't considered multiple viewpoints, thought about implications for practice, related issues to relevant theory, weighed up the evidence, etc., then you have not been fully reflective. Instead, you have remained superficial and descriptive. So all reflective writing should be critical.

It is easy to fall into the same traps as in academic writing, however. Make sure you explain everything. Draw out your points rather than leaving it to your reader to make their own conclusions. Consciously ensure you are taking a critical approach – to your actions and behaviours and to the topics that you are discussing.

There are plenty of opportunities to demonstrate your critical skills within reflective assessments. There should be critical analysis and discussion throughout. Don't wait until the section in which you relate issues to theory. In your introduction, you may wish to critically discuss the model you have chosen (why that one and not another, its strengths and weaknesses, why it is appropriate for these circumstances). You may even begin with a discussion of why reflection is important to the profession and the improvement of your professional practice. In the evaluation of your actions you could be critical by reflecting on how you felt at the time, immediately afterwards and now, in hindsight. There may be differences in how you feel about the incident and you could examine what might explain these. That is a much more complex task than simply writing about what the critical incident felt like at the time. You would be bringing in multiple perspectives – all yours, but at different distances from the event.

In your search for meaning, the critical skills you have developed through reading and evaluating research are important. If a particular theory seems relevant to your experience explain why this is the case. Do not simply accept the theory; look for evidence within the literature and examine how well the theory fits or helps you to understand your particular circumstances. If you are drawing upon published sources as evidence, evaluate them and write about their strengths.

Evidence within reflective writing

Since reflection concerns your experiences and feelings, some people become confused about when to use references and evidence. In fact, you should reference reflective work just as you would any other piece of formal, assessed writing. It is not necessary to provide evidence to prove that the incident happened or that you felt in a particular way about it. Nor can you do anything other than state how you think you performed or behaved. But, as we have discussed earlier, reflection is much more than the description of an event and the consideration of your feelings about it. Thus, in all other aspects of your writing, it is necessary to draw upon credible evidence to build your argument.

For some parts of reflection, once you have recognised that it is essential to provide references, it is reasonably straightforward to understand what kind of source you could use and where to place it within your writing:

- If you are introducing reflection, you can demonstrate its importance by referring to published work: '55 per cent of healthcare professionals in Roberts' study (2014) believed that reflection was one of the cornerstones of their practice. The North West NHS Trust (2011) argues that every newly qualified practitioner should set aside time each week to undertake critical reflection, such is its value.'
- If you wish to discuss the use of a particular model, again it is clear that you should provide a reference: 'I employed the Liddle (2009) reflective circle to facilitate my reflection. The five stages of the model have also been utilised to structure this essay.'
- When providing background detail, use published evidence to point your reader in the direction of further reading and to substantiate your claim: 'My role was to assist in training the client in how to take a reading from a peak flow meter. This device is used widely with people diagnosed with asthma (NICE, 2011, Feelty, 2013) and can be effective in …'
- When writing about your plans for future learning you might wish to directly refer to procedures you wish to master. 'Further understanding of the uses of hydrotherapy (Reid, 2009) will be invaluable, particularly in relation to spinal cord injuries (McGhie, 2013).'

For other elements of your reflective assessments, however, it is not quite so clear where you should draw evidence from. In these circumstances, it is a case of considering what theories/research/disciplines would help you understand the situation. You may have already covered the topics during your course (think back to earlier years and your psychology, sociology knowledge, for example) or perhaps you will have to research the issue from scratch as you would with any other assessment.

Activity: what kind of evidence?

Consider the following situations. Can you think of any areas of study or theory that might help inform a discussion? What kind of references/evidence might be useful?

1. Reread 'the presentation' extract above: nerves get the better of you during a presentation, you rush, miss things out and feel disappointed and frustrated with your performance.
2. Reread the 'group task' extract above. Your group is not working well together and some members do not seem to be working as hard as others.
3. Your critical incident concerns your relationship with your placement mentor. You feel that you are not being given enough responsibility and that, when you ask for support, your mentor simply takes over rather than supervising you or providing you with information to help you understand the situation better.

There are notes at the end of this chapter.

Hopefully, the tools and skills you have developed over the course of this book can help you take a critical approach to everything – from television programmes to professorial lectures, from government policy to research papers. Whether it is a reflective piece, a literature review or a case study, your approach should be the same. By asking questions, evaluating and analysing, building a logical argument and explicitly demonstrating your critical abilities in your writing you will be capable of thriving during the latter part of your degree and on, into professional practice.

Mistakes in reasoning

False cause

There must have been something wrong with that pint. I feel absolutely awful this morning.

The extra vitamins I'm taking definitely work. I haven't had a cold for months.

In both arguments, the person is attributing a cause to the result with no evidence or necessary logical connection. They blame the pint for their current illness or vitamin supplements for their current health. They may be correct but you would require further evidence to make such claims and there may be other possible explanations. Just how many pints were drunk, for example? Is it more likely that the person is hungover? Has the second person simply been lucky these last few months?

Notes on activity: evaluating reflective writing

The presentation

This extract appears to be an honest account that probes the participant's behaviour and feelings. It questions why things might have occurred as they did – running out of time, frustration that hard work was not demonstrated. The final action planning sentences are rather weak, however. What is going to make the person become 'less nervous'? This isn't something that happens simply because you hope it will. It is important that you are specific when planning – what exactly will you do to improve? How will you recognise when you have been successful in those endeavours?

The group task

This is quite a weak piece of reflective writing. There are a number of issues with the writing style – informal in places (tricky, if I am honest) and a little rambling. It is also far too descriptive with lots of details that do not add anything to our understanding. Do we need to know that it was the third module? If so, this should be made clear. Does the meeting venue (café) have any significance? Again, this would need to be explained to the reader. If not, it is irrelevant and can be left out. This would focus both the writer and the reader on the critical aspects of the reflection. What might explain the group dynamics? What could be done about it, for example?

Notes on activity: what kind of evidence?

There are no right or wrong answers for this activity. You may have ideas that I have not noted but this does not mean that they are without value. The aim is to search for meaning from the body of published knowledge. So long as you can make a logical link between the evidence and the topic, use it.

1.   Possible literature searches might focus on public speaking, performance anxiety, mindfulness and cognitive behavioural therapy, voice control.
2.   Evidence might be sought in the fields of group dynamics, non-verbal and verbal communication, role setting, inter-professional working.
3.   Your understanding might be broadened by investigating mentorship and supervision, professional confidence and becoming an independent practitioner, identity, difficult conversations.

Index